DRIVING FORWARDS

DRIVING
FORWARDS

A journey of resilience and
empowerment after life-changing injury

SOPHIE L. MORGAN

SPHERE

SPHERE

First published in Great Britain in 2022 by Sphere

1 3 5 7 9 10 8 6 4 2

A CIP catalogue record for this book
is available from the British Library.

Hardback ISBN 978-0-7515-8224-6
Trade paperback format ISBN 978-0-7515-8223-9

In order to maintain anonymity in some instances,
the author has changed the names of certain individuals.

Typeset in Garamond by M Rules
Printed and bound in Great Britain by
Clays Ltd, Elcograf S.p.A.

Papers used by Sphere are from well-managed forests
and other responsible sources.

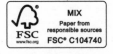

Sphere
An imprint of
Little, Brown Book Group
Carmelite House
50 Victoria Embankment
London EC4Y 0DZ

An Hachette UK Company
www.hachette.co.uk

www.littlebrown.co.uk

To Mum, Dad, Tom and Bowl,
and to ALL of the friends who have
got me by with a little help

I: THE BEFORE

The Road Scar

Hurtling along the road running parallel to a runway on an enormous three-wheeled motorbike, the speedometer creeping tantalisingly close to '100 mph', I take a deep breath and look towards the television camera that is dangling precariously out of the boot of the car in front of me. Its lens is fixed on my every move.

Taking one hand off my handlebars, I signal for the convoy to turn, and then to stop.

'So, *this* is where it happened?' the cameraman asks as he jumps out of the car, looking around as though there might be one of those roadside shrines, dead flowers and weathered teddy bears laid out. But there's nothing, just empty fields. That is, unless you know where to look. I nod back distractedly, searching the tarmac.

'Great! Excellent,' he says, repositioning his camera. 'Here we go! ACTION!'

His elation feels slightly inappropriate to me, a touch disrespectful, but I don't dwell on it – not because I'm impervious to insensitivity, trust me, this place is a minefield of emotion, but because at that moment my attention is elsewhere and I've just found what I was looking for, the only clue that this *is* the place: a deep semi-circular black slash in the tarmac.

The road scar smirks up at me, like an old friend who knows too many secrets. A remembrance of things past.

I nod back, out of respect, and hit the kill switch on my engine.

Looking around me expectantly, shivering slightly despite my bike gear protecting me from the cool wind coming from the North Sea only a mile away, I wait for the apparition of the Scottish policeman who found my body here the night the scar was carved into the road to appear. I'd been unconscious by the time he arrived but nevertheless, I have always pictured him vividly and I know now that somewhere deep down, I have carried with me the shock he must have felt at seeing my young, mutilated body, trapped upside down within the crushed frame of my car. My face split in half. My naked ass in the air.

But I do sometimes wonder if he may not have been all that surprised, and if maybe he had a more cynical reaction: *here we go again*, yet *another* young driver, naive to the danger she was in and with less than six months on her licence. *How predictable*, he might have thought, searching through the wreckage.

I assume that it was this very policeman who, having already dealt with the gruesome task of getting me and my friends out of the wreckage and into the ambulance, had the even more unenviable task of calling my poor parents.

Apparently, when the call came at four in the morning to tell them that their eighteen-year-old daughter and four of her friends had been involved in a car crash, the first thing Mum asked was if we all *walked* into the hospital. Isn't that a *brilliant* question? Of course, her training as a nurse helped.

But I should also tell you that when they explained to Dad – who recovered the phone after Mum had collapsed – that in fact I had *not* walked in, that I was in a 'critical condition', with extensive facial injuries and suspected 'spinal damage', Mum immediately cried, 'What level?' to which Dad repeated the answer through swallowed gulps. 'C6?' he told her. 'I think they said her C6 is damaged?'

Mum didn't tell Dad what that meant. That damage at that level of the spine could leave me paralysed from the neck down; she kept that to herself. It was at this point Mum decided that if I didn't die, she may have to kill me anyway.

Years later, when she told me this over a glass – let's be honest, a bottle – of wine, I laughed. Not a laugh that might suggest I agreed with that decision, but the despairing scoff of a person who knows that her mother, like so many people, presumed that disability of this kind could be a fate worse than death.

Perhaps it was having the maiden name of Fortune, and being called Miss Fortune – till she married my dad and became a Morgan – that made my mother so wary. Since I was old enough to remember, I'd been made to memorise the list of unfortunate conditions Mum deemed to justify euthanasia and what I must do if the worst were to happen to her. Firstly, don't tell anyone, *darling*, and then, simply, put a pillow over her head. As a former nurse she felt she had seen enough to be able to make an informed decision over her fate, whatever it might be.

It's apt, I think, that my mum named me after *Sophie's Choice*.

'Sophie?' the director shouts at me now. 'Are you okay?'

Snapping back into the moment, I see five pairs of eyes watching me and feel tension and concern hovering in the fresh spring air. Each member of the crew has expressed their reservations about our filming at the place where I so nearly died but, back then, in the planning-room in London, seven hundred or so miles south of this spot, in the well-practised tone I'd adapted to stave off any assumed fragility or fear on my part, I'd reassured them that it would be cool, I'd be *totally fine*, but I find people tend to doubt my conviction – for reasons I will come to explain. The truth is, I knew it would be good to be back. I had chosen to return.

When I first discovered the scar, eight years after it was created, I was also being flanked by a camera crew but unlike last time, I remind myself, straightening out my posture and clearing my throat, I haven't come back to find clues. This time, I am here for a different reason.

'Eighteen years ago,' I say clearly, looking into the camera, 'my life ended *just here.*' I glance down at the scar on the road. '*But* another life started and, today, I am back, at the beginning of my next chapter.'

The thrill these words give me is palpable. In the decade I've been presenting on television, I have never had my *own* series. I'm also unscripted and I feel liberated, a bit like being the only naked person in a room full of strangers. Which, coincidently, is also something I have actually done on TV, but we will get to that later.

For the purpose of the series I have been travelling around the UK, going to some extraordinary places and meeting some extraordinary people in order to learn about the radical changes they have made to their lives in pursuit of happiness and fulfilment, and to find inspiration for changes I intend to make to my life moving forward. The past year has been a particularly testing time, and the sense of achievement I feel being in front of the camera *and* riding my trike all the way to Scotland is almost overwhelming.

I look down at my weathered black biking jacket, worn in on the mission I've now completed, and it excites me to think how awful I must look. Normally, as a presenter, I'd be a veneered version of myself: hair tonged, make-up perfect. But today filth and grime from the motorways and back roads are splattered over me and my trike and these are the marks of achievement I haven't wanted to wash away. As the camera lingers on me, I remind myself to soak it up. *This is happening.* I have *made* it happen and it has taken me eighteen years to get here.

I yank off my helmet and let my long, tangled blonde hair fly where it wants.

The specially modified machine between my legs catches the sun and I hear the fan cooling the engine down. I got it as an eighteenth anniversary gift to myself, in order to feel as liberated as is physically possible for someone like me. And, sitting astride it, exposed to the elements, with so much power in my hands, having ridden to the summit of my wildest dream, at the place where one life ended, I wonder if it's possible to feel more alive.

Suddenly, from the Royal Air Force base beside us, a Typhoon fighter jet launches down the runway and off into the sky, screaming overhead, and in an instant, the sound takes me back to the very first time I strapped in behind the steering wheel of a car, with my breath held tight and my grubby teenage fingernails blanched white against the car key; I was gagging for the invitation to start the car's engine, when one of these fighter jets, chasing the wind that whipped through the clouds above, erupted over the top of my head. The car and I had trembled as the jet soared up and away and, before I could stop myself, before permission had been granted by the driving instructor, I twisted the car key and my foot pushed down on the accelerator, as though to follow the jet and take flight.

You see, for certain types of drivers, roads parallel to runways are seductive. Time it *just* right and the reckless among you will discover what I once did: that when you speed head-first foot-down along a road-cum-runway, you might feel as though you too can take off.

As long as you can get your damned car to go fast enough.

The more wary or cautious drivers among you, however, might know something that may take the rest of us years to learn: that these particular roads – like us particular drivers – can be the deadliest. Yes, learning to drive beside an Air Force base may well have confused my expectations, but the fact is the lessons required for me to get my driving licence came and went with absolutely no mention of the fact that a driving licence could potentially kill, and, accordingly, back then, it simply never occurred to me that in my hands, a life that was about to take off could instead come to an end.

When I drove down this road on that fateful night eighteen years ago, I was also about to embark on the long-awaited next chapter of my life. But I was distracted, blindsided by longing, giddy with anticipation for what was to come.

I look down to my disabled body, momentarily saddened, and imagine the road scar whispering up at me, *and look what happened to you.*

In the years since the crash, I have scoured the memory of that night with the ferocity of a pack of wolves scavenging a carcass. Blooded, I return conflicted, even now. You see, one part of me wants to clasp my eighteen-year-old face in my hands, pull her towards me and scream as loud as a fighter jet, so loud my throat tears, *Wake up,* girl. *LOOK out!*

But, looking back, what *would* I want to do differently? Would I warn her what was going to happen? Perhaps not, I think, my mind fizzing, the camera light still blinking. Perhaps I would say nothing at all.

Impulsive, childish and foolish, I now know there was no better way for her to go but forward, to drive head-first into the unknown. To fall forward into life. Because if she hadn't, then I wouldn't be where I am now, about to do exactly the same.

Last Photographs

Mum came north planning to smother me, unaware she was carrying with her the last photographs taken of me standing – and not just standing: in the freshly developed photographs tucked at the bottom of her handbag, her eighteen-year-old daughter was play-fighting and howling with laughter. On closer inspection, though, let me tell you, that girl was up to something. I was scheming something top secret. But watching me through the camera viewfinder, Mum wouldn't have suspected a thing.

We didn't know each other that well then.

The photographs were taken the day before the crash, on a disposable camera Mum remembered was at the back of that *sodding* kitchen drawer she could never fully close. Fussing through a tangle of wires, she retrieved it gleefully and rushed out into the garden, calling my brother and me into the sunshine with her. It was rare for us all to be at home at the same time and Mum said she wanted a keepsake before I left home, proof that she had done her job as a mum, evidence I existed once I had flown the nest.

Those were the days before camera phones, when developing disposable cameras tested Mum's patience. Today, thankfully, she doesn't have to endure the wait and I'd hazard a guess her mobile phone carries over a thousand photos of my brother and me, photos of photos even. Ever since that day, Mum keeps me with her at all times, on her person. Just in case.

Of the twenty-four photographs developed from that camera only a handful remain. I searched and searched but I gave up; most of the photos and the negatives are well and truly gone. Of the few that are left, four were framed and hung in my parents' home, but one, with its sharp corners now split open and curling back and holes pinpricked around the border, I keep with me, along with a photo of the photo (stored on the cloud in a folder named 'Dead'), so that I am on my person, at all times. Proof that I existed. Just in case.

Currently, the photograph itself is tacked to a board along with other sentimental miscellaneous crap beside business cards, Polaroids from parties, wedding invitations and scrap-paper with children's hands outlined, as though the person in the photo still exists in my chaotic life. A souvenir from the past.

But wherever or whenever I see the girl's face in the photographs, the truth is I no longer see *me*. Not by way of the fact that all of our younger selves look different, but because, as far as I am concerned – let me just flatten out the creases – yep, many of the features we once shared were destroyed.

Her face is symmetrical. The nose is straight and long. One eye socket matches the other in shape. Her young lithe frame stands supple, free from the pain and exhaustion of carrying a broken body, her shoulders look slack. Her thin arms are proportionate. Her smooth skin carries only the usual scars, the type that don't tell unusual stories. Scars from acne or learning to ride a bike, not the other sort that make people stare or elbow their friends to help them in a guessing game to work out *what do you think happened to her?*

The structure of her is as nature intended for her.

The bones protruding in her chest remind me of the skeleton

models that sat in a classroom corner during those lessons that taught us how human bodies are *meant* to work.

I used one of the photographs of her face as a reference for one of my paintings once, and when it was finished, I titled the painting *The Fool* because she was one, and I layered it in antique varnish, because she's now locked in the past.

Yes, I know, her mouth takes the same downward slope as mine, her brow bones cast the same shadow shapes and, yep, I am sure you won't agree with me but it's true: I just don't recognise myself in her. I am not the only one. *That's not you, is it?* people who didn't know me in the before ask, as they lean into my painting searching for clues.

But the highlight of white paint I dabbed on to the eye of the painting, that trickster's glimmer, that shimmer of her soul, that I recognise.

That came with me into this life.

There are others like me who recognise the dissonance between themselves before and after their injuries. It goes far beyond a curious confusion at seeing a person in the present and in their past, beyond the shock of a 'before and after' comparison. Seeing yourself before the trauma, before the change, feels both reassuring *and* unsettling. I wonder if it's one of the best *and* the worst types of nostalgia a person can manage. We all have versions of ourselves in the past that we miss, or that we wish to be forgotten, but what I am talking about is different. The more time I have spent writing about *her*, the more I find this to be true.

I'll begin by explaining that, in my experience, who you were as a person in the 'before' makes all the difference to who you become in the 'after'.

Our stories start at different times.

I will start with hers.

Her Story

When anyone asks what I was like *before* the crash (and oddly, they do, more often than you'd think), my mum will tell them that I was always *that* kind of girl.

The kind of girl who would give everyone else nits.

The kind of girl that loves trouble, hurtling full tilt towards it.

The kind of girl that would always get caught, get expelled. *That* sort.

Ill-fated is what she means. And she's not wrong.

She'd also tell you – unprompted – that I screamed *solidly* for the first three years of my life. I screamed and screamed, until the day a doctor realised I was allergic to the sap coming from the birch trees that surrounded our home, and to milk, which was alarming news given I had been lavishly doctored with the latter to try to soothe the former.

I'm no expert, but it would seem, therefore, any inner angst may have started before I was even conscious of it, along with a dangerous propensity for using ineffectual and harmful ways to self-medicate. Who knows? Whatever the long-term repercussions may have been, it was obvious early on that I would always be an irritant.

Thanks to an industrial amount of antibiotics, the wailing and excess mucus started to dry up, and eventually a short-lived peace reigned in our household – into which my brother was born, without *any* complications, Mum would add – and it was around then, after the rashes and swelling had gone down, that I was given my first chance to make up for all the trouble I had caused so far in my tiny life. I was scouted to be a child model. Mum was delighted; surely all the sleepless nights had been worth it? But the day before my first photoshoot, I got my squidgy little mitts on a pair of scissors and chopped off all my hair while Mum wasn't looking.

I wish I could tell you that this was the beginning of a style icon or the making of a future hairstylist, but it definitely wasn't. This was the first of several warning signs that, left to my own devices, I would most likely fuck things up. And by things, I mean myself.

The trees that I was allergic to belonged to Ashdown Forest, known round the world as The Hundred Acre Wood, home of the fictional character Winnie-the-Pooh, and we lived in the forest, in a cottage called Little Birches. With no neighbours in sight in any direction, the cottage had a fairy-tale feel about it. And while I, the anti-princess, may have had my own beautifully decorated little bedroom, with A. A. Milne's characters that Mum had painstakingly painted on the walls, hands down my favourite place to sleep was with the dogs, in the front porch, cuddled up with my best friend, Sumo, a yellow Labrador, permanently lathered in fox shit. I loved the way we would wake up still entwined, my own white-blonde mop tangled with her fur, feeling like I was an animal too.

Of all of my mum's animals – one horse, two cats and four dogs – Sumo was the only one that I was allowed to play (and sleep) with because, unlike her other dogs, Sumo was considered a pet, whereas the rest were what Mum called 'income'. I didn't know what that meant at the time, but whatever 'income' was, I didn't like it very much. It stressed everyone out. Mum

would swear at me if I played with the other dogs, especially if
I tussled at tug of war with them after Sumo had become tired
of me yanking her about the forest, snot streaming down my
face as I rubbed up against the birch trees. They were Mum's
'working' dogs, which she trained, and accordingly they had to
be treated with respect.

Despite my unquestionable loyalty to Sumo, as soon as my
mum's dog-whistle summoned her working dogs to her, I would
rush out of whatever bush I was tangled in and bolt back to
her feet, where I would *sit and stay* with the rest of them, Sumo
lolling around behind me. No matter how many dogs Mum had
under her command at one time, they'd all sit rigid like statues –
me among them, obediently playing along – the only give-away
we were alive, the whites of our eyes flashing as we watched her
every move, hardly daring to breathe without permission.

This was my mum in her element: waxed leather chaps over
faded denim jeans and a button-down shirt usually missing a
button, her hair scraped away in a braid so she wouldn't have to
bother washing it for at least a week, maybe more if she could get
away with it. In her lifetime, Mum had been a nurse, a midwife,
a stable groom, an air stewardess, a gun-dog trainer, a paper girl
and a pharmaceutical representative. I would one day come to
wonder what she might have been in another life, when women
weren't capped in their ambitions; Mum was a nurse, never a
doctor, a stewardess, never a pilot. Not that it mattered in my
mind; she was all things, everything and more. Perhaps because
of the societal barriers that prevented her from levelling up as a
woman in seventies Britain, Mum was determined to do what
she could to remove any barriers for me and she told me repeatedly I could be *anything* that I wanted to be in life but stressed
that it would be best *not* to have children. *They will ruin your
life,* she said plainly, as she hugged me so hard it tickled, and
I'd giggle, wondering what that meant exactly.

Mum was unquestionably the leader of our pack, looking after her animals and her children, which, by the way, was the order in which we were fed. Unless Dad was cooking, which, thankfully, most of the time he was. He did so not just because Mum refused to, but because Dad loved nothing more than being the 'host', bringing everyone together, and that meant the more food and wine, the better. Gregarious and fun-loving, Dad controlled all the fun (and the music) in our home. As a wine broker, he had a seemingly never-ending supply of wine, and so, tucked away in the forest where he could crank up the music, he and Mum would host parties every weekend and dance with their friends all night long, and my brother Tom and I would watch them from the bottom of the stairs through the crack in the door, laughing as they bopped away to M People, Eric Clapton, Simply Red, Right Said Fred and The Rolling Stones, cigarette smoke drifting over until we practically conked out from the fumes.

I spent my feral childhood wandering around the forest climbing trees and looking for Pooh sticks with Sumo and, when he was old enough to follow me, my brother Tom. In our world, being able to hide and seek was the only thing that mattered, and so every day, no matter the weather, our little legs would carry us up trees or into the bramble bushes, over streams and into muddy swamps. For hours Tom and I would trample through the forest, trying to out hide-and-seek each other, until the shadows started to frighten us, or Mum's dog-whistle called us back, and we would scamper home as fast as our mud-laden wellies would allow.

As children, if my brother or I were ever to leave the forest it would be either for something horse or dog related or to go to school. It took us about one play of the whole *Jagged Little Pill* to drive from the cottage to school, and en route, I honed some of my finest habits from the back seat, swearing being my favourite. *'I'm brave but I'm chicken-SHIT!'* I sang manically each morning, before Mum confiscated my Alanis Morissette tape. I learnt from the best, though: Mum's new best friend Sara, a powerhouse of a woman, swore so casually it was as though half of the English language came adjoined with a profanity. *You know fuckin-what?* Sara would say, *Carpe that fucking diem!* I had never met a more outspoken woman in my life and it left a significant impression on me. She laughed freely, talked loudly about politics and expertly about music and she did that thing I'd always been told not to do: she 'made a scene'. I quickly grew to love her as a second mother, and together with my own dominant outdoorsy and self-reliant mum, I began to shape in my mind the kind of woman I would like to be when I grew up. One that didn't *need* anyone, certainly not a man.

I understood the absence of their working husbands to mean they were independent women. It didn't occur to me that the two of them – both married, both mothers – were interdependent and that that kind of arrangement was perfectly acceptable, nor did it occur to me that dissuading me from having children or depending on a man was somewhat paradoxical, certainly hypocritical. I ingested their propaganda, and grew up bold, feisty, foulmouthed and headstrong, if not slightly confused.

I then discovered my two great loves. First, swimming. Nothing made me happier than the exhilaration of standing poised on the front of a diving board, my toes curled over the edge, waiting for the whistle to sound, flinging myself into the cool pool water, holding my breath for as long as I could as I rushed into whatever stroke we were racing, glancing at the other swimmers behind me before I reached out my hand and touched the wall first. I swam so much, chlorine seeped into me and if I licked my skin at any time, I could always taste and smell it. Dad called me his water baby. Mum hated the water and preferred me on a horse. To maintain the peace, I did both, and, to soothe the growing pressures of their expectations, I also learnt to shoot. There was something about knowing I was in control of something dangerous that made my little heart sing; to me using a gun was like using a swear word, shocking and emboldening, particularly when coming from a girl.

My second great love was art. My papier-mâché wine bottles were unusually convincing, apparently, along with my skill at capturing people's likeness in charcoal or landscapes in acrylics. One of my paintings was good enough to earn me an Art Scholarship to The King's School, Canterbury, and so, aged thirteen, I headed off to Big School. *It's time to fall in love*, I wrote in bold red pen in the new snazzy journal I had bought especially. *And hopefully get fingered!*

Thrown into a mixing pot with hundreds of other kids from all over the world, as a little country bumpkin I was in heaven. The classrooms were all spread around Canterbury city, at the heart of which stood an imposing but breathtaking cathedral. Each morning, bells would ring out and the eleven boarding houses and day houses across the city would spill open, sending sleepy students off to class. But I wasn't sleepy; I was wide awake, I could feel the pull of temptation in every direction: countless people to get to know, sports to try, teachers to outsmart – even the city itself seemed to be encouraging me to step out and explore.

At night from my dormitory bed, I could hear the pubs spilling out, glasses smashing, men catcalling and women retaliating. On the weekends, bass music from a neighbouring club made the single-pane windows reverberate. It was like I was sitting on the bottom step of the stairs again, eavesdropping on a party, but this time I was old enough to get involved.

All of my competitive and creative energies were repurposed: my goal to investigate and experiment. With my headphones on and music blaring, I started heading into the city to seek out the off-licences most likely to accept my fake ID, then grab as many other girls as possible and hide in the back alleys and towpaths of the city, testing out our limits with spirits, schnapps or the schoolgirl's champagne, Lambrini. My friends and I begged an older girl to teach us how to smoke, and in exchange for a week's worth of house duties, she snuck us into one of the bathrooms, locked the door, put a condom over the air vent and a rolled-up towel underneath the door, and cranked open all the windows. Handing us each a cigarette and a lighter, we got through a packet in less than half an hour, threw up, and then started all over again. I was hooked.

But, as Mum says, I am as subtle as a heart attack.

The school caught on to my bad behaviour and I was sanctioned, making it impossible for me to play my teenage version of hide-and-seek in the city any more. Letters went out to my parents telling them of my behaviour but, thankfully, being at boarding school meant I didn't have to look either of them in the eye.

When the summer came around, like an escaped convict I returned to the forest only to dart out into the closest town. With both my parents out at work, I took off to the streets of Tunbridge Wells with some pals and made up for lost time.

In the park, with my local friends, taking turns on a vodka bottle like suckling pigs on a teat, pissed and unsupervised, we rolled around on the grass, crying with laughter, belting out Oasis songs and making up dance routines to 5ive. One afternoon, as I rushed to get home, I drunkenly mistimed alighting the bus, and knocked myself out on the bus stop. I came to with Mum dragging me by my hair into the back of her car, wherein she sped back to the forest and sobered me up by lunging me in circles like a horse around the garden, exercising the booze out of me. Earlier that week I had tried to hide more evidence of my underage drinking by lobbing some wine bottles stolen from my dad's cupboard into the bracken behind the house, but Mum's work dogs retrieved them, like informants plonking them at the front door of the house. *Traitors*. Old Sumo had my back, of course, trundling behind me as I weaved, pissed, around in circles in the garden, but to everyone else, it was obvious I was losing my way.

When I returned to school for the start of the second year, I was on thin ice. In an attempt to prevent any further bad behaviour, my house mistress decided to 'gate' me indefinitely. Unable to leave the boarding house for any reason other than classes or meals, I was indefinitely 'locked down'. I was beyond enraged; honestly, hell hath no fury like a vindictive privileged British schoolgirl. The school should have predicted that stricter sanctions for my wayward behaviour would not reduce any chance of recidivism.

I decided to take action.

After all, 'gated' didn't actually mean I was *locked* in, just *forbidden* to leave the house, so when no one was watching I snuck through the back gate, having elicited the code out of an unwitting newspaper delivery man. Poor man had no idea what he'd done.

I went on the rampage. I had worked out a way to carry contraband in the lining of my long black trench coat, so after purchasing several litre bottles of vodka, I slipped them into their hiding place and headed out to meet my friends in the city.

But when I got caught a few hours later, it was obvious my 'plan' had not been as cunning as I'd hoped. The school had caught me on CCTV pacing down the high street in my full-length black trench coat and sunglasses and suspended me (and my friends) immediately.

I returned to the forest, embarrassed and ashamed of my stupidity. I couldn't even look Sumo in the eye. Mum and Dad barely spoke to me for the entirety of my seven-day suspension and to make matters worse, the school called to tell them my house mistress would no longer take me back and as no other boarding house would either, an unprecedented decision had been made. I would have to sleep in the school's sickbay. My mouth fell open as though I was expecting my tonsils to be examined.

But something about my behaviour being unrivalled in its awfulness felt like an achievement. No other student in the school's long history had been exiled in this way. What an adventure! I didn't even know where the sickbay was, having never needed to go there before, and I pictured something not too dissimilar to the psychiatric hospital in *One Flew Over the Cuckoo's Nest,* and myself as the rowdy but lovable flouter-of-rules. Like McMurphy, I would stick it to the institution!

When I returned to school a week later, I returned notorious, and the reward for my outstanding unruliness? I finally got my first boyfriend. He asked me to 'go out with him', and as soon as I had nodded yes with the dumb enthusiasm of a slobbery dog, he yanked me towards him and plunged his tongue into my mouth. Friends around us cheered. Our mouths clamped together, our tongues wet and rapid, like a tumble dryer on a spin. As the chant of 'snog her, snog her' climaxed around us, I felt a pulse pound between my legs and when he let me go, the blood seemed to have drained out of my limbs. I stumbled back against a wall, dazed but delighted, in a disorientated stupor. *Alcohol has nothing on kissing,* I scribbled frantically in my diary, as though I had discovered the meaning of life, pressing my friends for more details on what third base was like, scared I wouldn't survive the ordeal, I would just keel over from a pleasure overdose.

My behaviour started to improve, so much so that, against all odds, I was allowed to go on a school trip to Spain. Things were definitely looking up.

But, out of the six girls who were caught drunkenly running riot around central Seville only twenty-four hours into the school trip, there was only one who was sent home. No prizes for guessing who. Whoever it was that told me that sucking on a copper penny would stop a breathalyser from working was either out to get me or was as gullible a son of a bitch as I was.

I got busted *and* practically choked to death. I was then asked, in no uncertain terms, to leave the school, and never come back.

After that, Mum threatened to *pack it all in and emigrate to Australia.* Dad muttered *disappointment* at me whenever he could look at me. And no other school would take me. Until one day, Sara called to tell my parents about a school she knew of in Scotland, and over the phone I picked up the words 'unique' and 'isolated', and the phrase that really grabbed my attention: 'character-building'.

What on earth did that mean? My school reports said I had *too much* character; surely building *more* character would be ruinous. But I didn't ask questions or put up a fight. I'd had enough of me and my ways, just as much as everyone else. I'd let everybody down, including myself. Thankfully, my brother helped me see the wood for the trees. Following in my footsteps, three years behind me, he told me without meeting my eyes that he was being humiliated by bullies in his class and my 'reputation' was hurting and embarrassing him. Mortified, I hugged Tom and apologised, looking his little round face square in the eyes, and I promised to do better, and to be better.

'Besides,' I told him optimistically, 'going to Scotland could be just what's needed to sort me out? I can't get any worse ...'

The decision to send me north wasn't an easy one for my parents to make. Even with another Art Scholarship, they could barely afford the fees and we wouldn't get to see each other very often, but the idea of me getting away from the temptations of the south and into the Highlands was what convinced my mum it would be worth their grafting for. Her father was Scottish, and Mum believed a reconnection to the Motherland could be good for me, a return to the wild.

Or at least that's how it felt as I belted myself into the long green itchy tartan kilt of the school uniform and journeyed to Scotland, into my next chapter.

Welcome to Scotland

Y anked away from my southern friends and, worst of all, any phone signal, I arrived in the Highlands of Scotland, initially a cold and unwelcoming environment. A Royal Air Force base to the east, a tiny fishing village to the south, rugged Morayshire coastline to the west, and the rest being the tempestuous North Sea, my new school felt to me as though it had been entirely forgotten, rejected by the rest of the world. A bit like I'd been. The school buildings were crumbling and sodden, and the staff appeared as weathered as the clifftops on which the school stood. Everything looked tired of fighting with the elements, everything looked utterly fed up. And, 'no', the grey-skinned taxi driver explained, as he dropped me at the school gates, 'the nearest toon is aboot two hoors walk fae here, so ya cannae "pop" anywhere, ya dafty'.

Right then, that's me told. Or at least I think it is? I could barely understand what he had said.

Adjusting to my new school, I felt guilty for the trouble I had caused my family so was motivated to avoid upsetting them again. I wanted to start figuring out ways to work harder, and play smarter, and I wanted to make new friends, join new teams and, most tempting of all, get under some kilts . . .

But looking around me at the wooded empty grounds and

grey rain-stained Portakabins, I didn't feel very inspired. I didn't get a very warm reception from the students either. Stories about my arrival midway through the year were so speculative, many of the girls seemed to want to keep me at arm's length, just in case. I wasn't upset about this; I mean I got it, no one likes a mysterious blonde girl arriving without any warning, completely messing with the hierarchy. I was too surly to be approachable and too English to be welcome. But it made me long to leave, and I began to regret all my rebellious behaviour.

At the end of my first week, I was standing by myself, as a stream of students left classes for a mid-afternoon break, when a boy who I recognised from my maths class caught my attention and waved for me to come over. I ran towards him gratefully and introduced myself. He tapped two fingers against his mouth, as though kissing a peace sign. But this was not a peace sign. This was a trouble sign. This was the signal for 'do you want to come for a cigarette?' or in other words, *here we go again*.

I pushed out my lower lip, raised my eyebrows, turned over my palms, shrugged one shoulder up towards my head, and all together those gestures could only mean one thing: *Fuck it. Why not?*

My first Scottish pal, Jamie, started nattering away about the lay of the land. Thrilled to have made a new friend, I listened closely but then started to feel confused; we seemed to be following a stream of students straight into the woods. As we got to the treeline, I braced myself: what was I going to find in there? Jamie went first. Glancing around nervously, I followed him. It took a few seconds for my eyes to adjust to the dark and then a few more seconds to believe what I was seeing. Littered around the forest, in threes or fours, students were lighting up cigarettes. Groups of girls were sharing lighters, older boys were rolling and passing around tobacco papers, younger students stuck together, chugging and coughing, some were playing and some were climbing trees. As far as my eye could see, countless little red dots, the cherries of all the cigs, danced as though the trees had fairy lights in them. Jamie popped a lit cigarette in my mouth and I took a long, lovely drag. But where were the teachers? Smoking wasn't permitted. Even by my standards, no one was being at all subtle.

Then suddenly a cry of 'BASHER!!' echoed around the school grounds. As if being directed to freeze-frame by a drama teacher, all the students stopped what they were doing.

I had no idea what this meant but from the worried looks on everyone's faces it couldn't be good. Panic stricken, I grabbed Jamie's arm and pleaded for him to help. *I can't move to Australia!* I cried. But there was no need to panic; everyone knew exactly what to do.

Dropping all contraband, they fled. I followed Jamie, who did his best to explain as we ran that the cry signalled an infiltration of the groundskeepers who were called 'Bashers'. They routinely patrolled for smokers, drinkers, and any other banned behaviour in the woods that surrounded the school. Running low, so as to avoid the sweeping flashlight that was scouring the trees, the trick, he whispered as we stopped behind a tree, was to keep down and never stop moving and always, no matter what, run in formation, putting the fastest and preferably largest kid at the front so as to clear a path for everyone behind them to safely exit the woods and return to permitted grounds, thereby escaping punishment, which ranged anywhere from detention to outright expulsion.

This wasn't a game for the faint-hearted: recreational smoking was like a full-contact sport. One time, Jamie told me as we army-crawled through the woods to safety, a Basher rugby-tackled a boy to the ground, knocking his cigarette clean out of his mouth. Another time, one of the Bashers, chasing a particularly stealthy team of sixth-form girls, mistimed his speed and ran into the school lake.

It was as though the school was a battleground and the woods belonged to the students, like lost boys in Neverland, and no matter what the teachers tried to do to win them back, the tree-houses, underground dens and naughtiness, he said, would just evolve, getting more creative and elaborate every year.

'So, is this what they mean by character-building?' I asked Jamie jokingly when we'd exited the woods to safety.

'Aye,' he laughed. 'Welcome to Scotland.'

Within a few months, I started to settle in. I'd befriended the art teacher and decided to let him help me become the best artist I could be. Next, I tried out for the netball team and became the youngest girl in the school to be in the Firsts, which thankfully helped me to make some girlfriends.

The school appeared to believe in me and so I decided to turn over a new leaf and apply myself. But unfortunately, children like me are hard to change. No school could have protected me from myself; the only way I would learn anything would be the hard way or not at all. Like all of the other students who were to become my friends, I thought rules were meant to be broken just as roads next to runways were made for racing.

Winter arrived and with it never-ending snowball fights.

During one particularly ferocious battle between two of the boarding houses, a stray snowball hit me in the face, and before I knew it, one of the older boys was running at me. I took off, straight into the trees, hurtling through the snow. Glancing round, I saw the boy hadn't slowed down and was sprinting after me. I hurried on, laughing, and scooped up some snow as I went, pummelling it into a ball as I darted through the woods, but when I turned to throw it, I couldn't see him. Then, out of nowhere, he shot through the trees and caught me, knocking me clean off my feet. Writhing and thrashing on the ground underneath, I tried to get away but we made eye contact. Both of us stopped wriggling. His eyes – an intense dirty-brown with flecks of green – were fixed on mine. Up close this boy was intimidatingly handsome; he had thick dark eyebrows and a rounded rugged face shadowed by stubble, and thick, chapped lips which, I thought lustfully, looked to me as though they needed licking. Apart from my pounding heartbeat and panting breath, I was frozen still. He smiled to break the ice and instantly I did the same, and then, we kissed. It felt to me as though our lips fitted together like puzzle pieces; my hands untangled from his grip and I wrapped them around to hold the back of his head and pulled him hungrily closer to me. He slipped his hands under my jumper, I flinched at the cold, but we didn't stop. I opened my eyes as he kissed me and saw snowflakes had settled on his eyelashes. The boy and I were like two figurines inside a snow globe, just the two of us and the pine trees.

By the time spring came around, I'd fallen head over heels in love with him.

Truth be told, I had never felt so infatuated with anyone in my life, nor so attracted. Rory, a snowboarding skater type, was a year older than me and a head taller, and had a deep Scottish accent which could set off an avalanche in my knickers. It was as though he had invisible magnets in his hands that could pull me, crotch-first, towards him from any distance. I was dumbstruck with love. Every day before lessons, he'd saunter up behind me, wrap his hands around my waist, plant a kiss in the nook between my neck and shoulder, and we would walk with an earphone in each of our ears connecting us together like a vein, playing 'The Light' by Common on repeat.

He lived locally, around the corner from the school, down a long straight road that ran parallel to the RAF runway.

Before he went home every day, he'd meet me after lessons,

and we'd slide into the woods and coil up together in the grass, listening to music for hours. Most of the time, he was brooding and exhaustingly patriotic (his ability to see past my Englishness was deemed a testament to his love for me), but that made it all the more rewarding when I made him crack a reluctant smile or crease with laughter. I was addicted to him, and nothing could ever get me close enough to him, even when I was pressed up against him; even then, I wanted more of him. It was as though I could never be satisfied; my carnality was a bottomless pit I desperately needed him to fill.

But capricious and fickle, my sex drive took a sudden U-turn, and I swerved towards the forbidden, crashing into the arms of his best friend, Jack. Rory was abandoned.

In time, Rory forgave Jack for the betrayal, as though it was to be expected that as best friends they would share one another's possessions; I was no different to a well-fitted beanie or brand-new skateboard. *Clearly men have different metrics for friendships,* I thought, baffled – but relieved – as I watched them kick-flipping together outside the maths block a year later. But, no matter how many mix tapes I made him, Rory refused to forgive me.

Ill-fated as ever, though my greedy duplicity would not go unpunished.

'Have you heard about the local driving instructor with the red BMW?' Jack asked me as we sat side by side at the back of our English class, the summer after we turned seventeen. We had been inseparable from the moment we had stolen a kiss in the art block toilets behind Rory's back a few years earlier. Only a month apart in age, we had both been thinking about starting our driving lessons. I was desperate to get moving, desperate for the freedom that came with driving.

Our classroom door swung open lazily, flapping on the warm summer breeze. 'I heard that if he likes you, he'll let you do the drive-thru at McDonald's', Jack continued. Listening intently, I fingered the packet of ten Lucky Strike cigarettes hidden in the lining of my school jacket. '*And* I heard he lets you smoke in the car after your lesson.' I looked at him excitedly, and decided there and then, this was the driving instructor for me.

Outside, overhead, a pair of Typhoon fighter jets rocketed skyward; their noise rumbled in the distance, like a tropical storm approaching.

Inside, underneath our school desk, Jack fiddled with a rip in my black school tights, fingering at the hole to get through to the skin of my squidgy inner thigh. He tore the hole wider, and I moved my leg closer to let his hand slip inside. He squeezed me playfully then shuffled his chair closer to mine. He leant over and nibbled my left earlobe.

'Absolute no brainer really, isn't it?' I said as I opened my legs further so his hands could explore a little higher. Jack's fingers crept up into the heat between my legs. I looked around to see if anyone was watching but no one could see. Besides, the class knew better than to look our way when we took the corner seats. I shifted my hips on my seat, so that he could reach me more easily. I pulled out a pencil and began doodling on my textbook as a cover. Jack reached me and started to rub his thumb gently on me, around and around, in circles. Minutes later, my pencil marks began to trace the same shape, the dark swirl on the paper intensifying with every rotation. Jack, sitting upright to avoid being caught, continued: 'Yeah, and he's meant to be a really sound guy and,' he bent back over to me and whispered, 'he's very good ... at ... what ... he ... does.'

Looking down, I could see the ligaments in his hands flex in time as he spoke. I struggled to hold my pencil properly. *Christ.* I gripped the desk and bit my lip.

'Doing okay there, Soph?' His cheeky sexy Scottish lilt did nothing to help calm me down. 'You look a little *flustered.*'

'You know what,' I said, breathing out, finally, 'how about we make a little bet?' I felt his hand stop. 'I bet I'll pass my test before you?' I snapped my thighs closed and trapped his hand, then leant over to bite his right earlobe. 'What do you think?!'

Disappointed, he kissed me on the forehead. 'I don't want to *bet*, Soph, let's just take our time, pass when we're ready?'

'Okay, fine.' I rolled my eyes. He knew I would still try to beat him regardless. 'I can't wait to get started . . . Imagine, learning to drive in a fuckin' *Beamer*!'

Later, back at my boarding house, a group of girls were gathered around the seating area reserved for sixth-form girls. It was six thirty in the evening, everyone was meant to be in their rooms doing homework, but I scoured the room: as far as I could tell there were no adults kicking about to tell us off, so I squeezed through the crowd to find a seat and check out what all the fuss was about. The group of girls were laughing (some not altogether too kindly), and many were clapping along.

I looked to my friend Celia, who gestured for me to hurry up and pointed into the centre of the seating area where a tall, slim girl, with legs like a 1920s showgirl, was dancing wildly around in circles, her grey school skirt tucked into her tights, whooping and yelping as though she was at a Scottish ceilidh, and at the same time, playing an imaginary trumpet through the side of her mouth. I scoffed, but then joined in the clapping.

The girl, who had straight blonde-brown hair that fell around her shoulders – or it would have if she ever stood still – had a cherubic face and was sweating and spinning and attempting to run and tap dance up the wall. As we watched her showing off so shamelessly, I dropped my school bag.

'Who's she?' I said as I sat down next to Celia.

'I think her name's Antonia,' she replied. 'She's one of the new sixth-form kids.' Celia shrugged and we laughed.

The girl collapsed into a chair to catch her breath. Half of the crowd erupted in applause. I went over to introduce myself. 'Heya, I'm Sophie. Are you a dancer or something?' I said, but she wasn't interested in answering my question.

'Shall we go for a cig?' she said instead. *Do any kids at this school not smoke?* I thought despairingly. 'And can we take Sophia and Ellie? They're new like me. SOPHIA!' Antonia shouted as though she owned the place, and out of the crowd came a curly-haired girl with enormous owl-round eyes and an eager expression that read, *Whatever you're up to, count me in.* Sophia beamed expectantly at us both. And then another girl appeared, her hands on her hips like Peter Pan. Eye to eye with me while I was perching on the armrest of Antonia's chair, she must have only been about five foot tall but something about her tits-forward stance told me she would be able to kick my lanky ass, no bother. Strong and slender, with platinum-blonde hair, a Cheshire cat smile and several piercings in her ears, she said, 'Heya, I'm Ellie. Shall we go somewhere?'

Did I know then that these three would become my best friends, and that our friendship would one day help save my life?

Of course not.

But I had my suspicions.

Finally, I reached the last term of school.

Antonia – known by us as Boner or Bone – Ellie, Sophia and I were revising for our exams in the suntrap at the back of the boarding house, lying spread-eagled in the sun in our underwear, slathered in baby oil to help us catch a tan in the searing Scottish sun.

The final school dance was happening that evening, and sweating and excited, we put our books away and went up to get into the superhero costumes we'd been preparing over the last few days. It was only a matter of weeks till our exams and then school would be over.

I had recently turned eighteen, and I had also aced my driving test, passing first time, and ever since, a feverish urgency had grabbed hold of me: I was counting down the seconds until I was free. Free from rules and timetables. Free to be an adult.

I was hardly sleeping at night, I had been fretfully tossing and turning, soaking my bed sheets in sweat; the nights and days were dragging, it was hot and I was restless.

I caught eyes with a younger girl who was watching us out of her bedroom door.

I've done my time here, I thought. *I'm ready for what's next.*

Thanks to my holiday job working in a local pub, I had put away enough money to book a flight to visit my school friend Vaibhav at his home in India. My life was about to elevate; soon I would go where I wanted and be who I wanted. I was ready to be unstoppable.

'Everyone . . . ' Ellie said, interrupting my daydreaming, sitting up and pulling on her school uniform again, squinting at us in the sunshine. 'There's something that I have been meaning to tell you all, but you have to *promise* me you will all be nice about it?'

The three of us gave our word with a quick nod.

'I have a new boyfriend . . . ' And before we could say a thing she added, 'We met in the holidays and well . . . he's disabled.'

No one said anything. To me, the word disabled was pejorative and terrifying. It implied difference and, without question, otherness, inferiority and most paralysing of all, incapability. Tumbleweed may as well have rolled past us.

'Ellie . . . ' I mumbled as an image of a vulnerable, weak, pitiful disfigured boy sitting alone, in need of help, developed in my mind. 'You better not hurt him,' I said to her sternly. Then I paused and I asked, 'Wait, El . . . can he even have sex?'

*

Just like the scar in the tarmac on the road, this conversation is unerasable and haunting for me, and it holds clues that reveal deep, dark, dirty truths about the ableist attitudes I held and the person I once was.

It's unsurprising but nevertheless upsetting, therefore, that when the time came that I was to eventually meet a disabled person for the first time, I would meet them with this same ignorance, prejudice and soft bigotry, and unfortunately for me, the first disabled person I would happen to meet would be me.

Never Seen Again

My friends and I didn't blame the superhero costumes, but with hindsight, we admitted to one another as we left the headmaster's office the morning after the last dance, heads hanging low, they weren't the best idea.

'I think we let them go to our heads, didn't we?' I said.

Back in my room, we all sat down on my bed. I closed the door. Boner started gnawing at her fingernails. Soph hugged a pillow, expressionless. Ellie stood up and threw up in the bin.

'Oh well,' I kept on, the only one able to formulate a sentence, but I was rambling shite. 'At least we went out with a bang . . .'

My words fell flat. Ellie gagged again.

In the early hours of that morning, we'd been caught trashing the boarding house. Just as a plastic kettle hurtled past my head and smashed against a wall, our house mistress had walked in and found us, in bras, pants and capes, surrounded by destruction, and with that, it was game over.

The headmaster had just confirmed it. We had been asked to leave.

Thankfully, so close to our final exams, the school decided to let us sit them and not throw our futures out the window, like we had done with most of the common-room furniture.

I took my A levels a few weeks later and that was it, I was done.

School was over, and so off I ran into the summer. Planning and hoping to never look back.

Two months, or eight weeks, or fifty-six whole days later, I had just got back from India, and was busy dancing around in my bedroom in my pants to Faithless and Underworld, sorting out weeks of dirty washing and deciding where to hang my new drapes, when my phone buzzed and an unexpected name flashed up on the screen.

Rory.

I picked it up. The familiar lilt of his voice was enough to make my knees buckle. The way he sounded my name, that soft drop of the 'So', transported me straight back, so close to his mouth I could practically feel the puff of breath leave him as his lips parted ever so slightly at the gently exhaled 'phie'.

'There's a party tomorrow night, in the village next door to school. Are you coming up?' he asked.

'Yes,' I said immediately, even though I hadn't planned to. I was thinking of calling my school for my exam results instead of heading back to Scotland to collect them in person. But if he was going to be there, I was going. With the little money I had left over after the summer holidays, I booked a trip north.

The last time Rory and I had spoken there hadn't been a clean goodbye and, whether he knew it or not, as far as I was concerned, he and I had some unfinished business. Loose ends to close. Bottomless pits *to fill*. For me, therefore, an unexpected invitation north to see Rory was like one of those runway roads: so seductive I just had to take it.

Also, Jack and I were about to break up. We had both admitted to one another that it was probably time to end things and go our separate ways, now that school was over. That was just what was meant to happen at that time: the chapter was closing and so must our three-year relationship. Jack would be at the party so maybe it was best I go, to end it with him and then try to get with Rory, I thought, my concupiscent scheming mind going into overdrive.

I hung up the phone just as I heard Mum calling me downstairs so that she could take some photos of my brother and me. Mum snapped away at us both – howling with laughter and play-fighting in the garden – until the disposable camera ran out of photos.

Seconds after Mum took what became known as the 'Last Photos', I shot inside, taking the stairs two or three at a time, darting straight to her wardrobe to find some shoes for the party in Scotland. Being so tall, I would never have dreamt of wearing heels before, but I asked myself, what would a *woman* wear? What would *Sharon Stone* wear?

I approached the search like I would a game of netball. I identified a team of suitable players from Mum's selection and lined them all up for practice, trialling one pair after another by walking around Mum's bedroom, putting them through their paces: strutting, skipping, squatting and jumping. (When it comes to Scottish ceilidhs you can never be too prepared.) If my ankles didn't collapse and the shoes remained on my feet, they made the team. After twenty minutes of further trial and error, I finally selected the perfect pair. Black, pointed, with a covered toe and open back – which could prove potentially dangerous, but they had aced the jump and twist test – and, crucially, only a wee kitten heel. Looking at myself in the mirror as I slipped into the winning pair and rose up to a full six foot, I felt as though I was stepping into womanhood.

Mum walked into the room and into our reflection.

'Darling girl, you look so beautiful, all grown up.' Side by side we stood together. 'I'm so excited for you, Sophie. Getting your exam results, going off to university. This really is the start of the rest of your life.'

The next day Mum drove me to the station. Slowly and deliberately marking the significance of the moment, we hugged, and she wished me all the luck in the world for my exam results. All of it. Every little bit of luck there was. There was nothing subtle behind her drawn-out squeeze, nor in my pulling away.

'Love you, Mum,' I threw carelessly at her. 'I'll call you later.'

I hate to say this, but I don't think I even looked back.

I have no memory of what happened during the *day* of 17 August 2003. The last day I walked is a date that I have marked in my calendar ever since and yet I never know quite what to do with myself when it comes around. Most of the anniversaries are a drunken blur, which is ironic, given that on the evening of the date in question, nothing was drunken, or blurred.

My memory is crystal clear from the moment I arrived at the party.

Ducking into the toilets, I looked at myself in the mirror. I knew that my body had grown over the summer, or perhaps I had finally fully grown into it, and in preparation for the night ahead I'd shaved off my pubic hair and was going commando underneath my black dress, a hard white tan line from my bikini sliced across my hips, clean and perfect, ready to be made dirty. The dress hung down to my thighs, long enough not to have to worry about exposing too much when dancing, but short enough to pull off some *Basic Instinct* moves if I chose to do so – which, given my mood, I *totally* was. My long hair was white-blonde at the front and a deep honey brown down my back. I'd always disliked my lower body: my legs were dispro-portionate to the rest of me, thicker and chunkier, and for years I would try to cover up with a jumper wrapped around my bum, and loose baggy flares (in those days the less shoe you could see, the better). But today I felt differently.

Earlier that day I'd learned that I'd collected enough grades to get my place to read Law at Manchester University. I'd made it by the skin of my teeth, and the world was mine for the taking. Carpe that fucking diem, as Sara would say.

Satisfied with the way I looked, I went outside to have a cigarette.

And there he was.

Leaning on a car like a film star, Rory was looking out at the view, a rolled cigarette smouldering in his hand. If I had had any conflicting feelings about wanting to be with him when Jack and I were not quite over, they evaporated instantly. Just as they had years earlier, thoughts of the consequences of betrayal – this time to Jack – didn't sit long with me. I had heard rumours that Jack had cheated on me over the summer. *We have loved and hurt each other the same, and it will all be over soon,* I thought. The fresh start was around the corner. I just had this *one* last itch to scratch. After all, wasn't life just one big experiment in how much I could get away with?

In that part of Scotland, the vistas are enormous, uninterrupted and limitless, and so far north, the summer days are endless. In front of us the horizon spread out wide, with the full low August sun exposed and pulsating at its centre. Magic hour was upon us. The sky was electric, soaked in pink. The floral waft of my sticky-sweet perfume, with an undertone of pheromone, reached Rory before I did, and he turned, and smiled.

The number of times I have replayed this next move in my mind is beyond obsession. Each and every time I recall how I walked towards him, my heart lifts and breaks a little more. Over time this memory, like that old photograph, has somewhat creased, it has got a bit battered and maybe after eighteen years some details have changed or been forgotten. But after all this time, I have never let go of it. It is pinned longingly and painfully at the forefront of my mind.

I'll play it again now.

There I was, doing my best to high-heel my way towards him without falling, lapping up his gaze like a thirsty animal. Underneath the dark hood of his eyebrows, his eyes scanned every contour of my body.

'Whoa,' he said. 'You look different.'

Relieved to have made it in one smooth strut, I leant against the car, so close to him that the hair on our forearms touched. I rolled a cigarette. Running the goddamn world.

That was me.

Wait there, I might just play it again, just one more time.

You know those looks that speak a thousand words, the looks that speak to your body, to your heart, and tell you loud and clear without a sound that you are being enjoyed? Better still, devoured? Those specific gazes have the power to transform the way you move, like a puppet on a string. When someone looks at you a certain way, you become simultaneously conscious of yet completely out of control of your body. Like an animal who senses a presence, the hair on your neck rises up and you sharpen your posture in preparation to run either straight at or far away from the watcher.

I have never been a man, but I was once a young non-disabled woman, and I can tell you these silent exchanges are for their eyes only.

In my experience, men do not look at disabled women in that way.

That girl has gone and that would be the last time anyone saw her.

Driving away from the party that night with Rory, Jack, my friend Celia and Rory's younger brother in the car, I raced along the dark country lanes to our after-party and to what I hoped would be the final part of my fantasy – into Rory's bed. He was in the passenger seat and we were squabbling over music; I could feel Jack kicking me through the back of my car seat trying to get my attention. Celia and Rory's brother were singing, joyfully and drunkenly.

I flew down the runway road, past the RAF base.

The car raced at the speed of my lustful mind.

Missing the corner, I lost control of the steering, and hitting the verge the tyre burst, its rim slicing into the tarmac. And then the car took off into the field, flipping relentlessly before crashing down into the dirt, leaving behind a deep scar on the road.

Salty, gritty earth mixed with a tangy stinging taste of iron filled my mouth. One eye, blinking blindly, soaked in blood. I heard only one voice and I thought that it said *I love you*. I didn't know then what I had done to myself and how close I was to death.

All that mattered was him, and how close I was to having him. Then I guessed I must be upside down, and, if so, well, had my dress fallen down, and, wait, fuck, *what* was on show from underneath . . . ? *This is going to take a long time*, I thought.

Rushed to hospital, everything I knew was left behind. Even my mum's shoes.

I had no concept of where I was or of what had happened, and to try to explain where I believed I was would be to test your understanding of reality, challenge your beliefs on what happens when a human body and soul separate.

Simply put, I was somewhere else, where other people aren't. It was as though every nerve in my body was trying to get my attention, screaming at me to send help, but the noise was so overwhelming, I didn't know where to start. My focus was pulled in what felt like a thousand different directions. A sharp biting sting from what I assumed was my eye socket, a deep pulsating thud from where my nose might be, a stiff swollen ache in my jaws, my mouth so parched the gums had cracked, and the bitter taste of iron and vomit filling my mouth.

But more unnerving than all of that was the void I felt below me.

Where was the rest of me?

II: THE AFTER

My Story

The blood in my mouth was thick with grit and ground-up segments of my face. I spluttered and choked and tried to open my eyes, but only one slit of my left eyelid responded. The light was blindingly bright. I slammed it closed again. Everything felt upside down, and inside out. *Was it daytime? But where did the night go? Where did my life just go?*

Nurses rushed around me, screaming instructions. They counted down from three and then there was a flickering agony in my back. 'Will I still be able to have babies?' I said. Or tried to – the words were blocked by my split, swollen tongue. Blood spilt out of my mouth. My jaw, like a drawer that had been yanked open too quickly, seemed to have come off its hinges; it dangled to the left of me. I hissed and spat and choked again.

My head rolled backwards as though it was about to separate from the rest of me, my vision followed up towards my skull. Vomit trickled down from my mouth into my upturned nose.

The one eye closed and I passed out.

Sleep felt as though it came for me and kidnapped me from reality, taking me into a fever dream where my life was torn up into fragments. The sound of crushing metal and glass shattering. *Did someone say I love you? Where are the others?*

In my dreams a figure was waiting for me, it was leaning against the side of a car with a cigarette, it ran at me, grabbed my hair then smashed my face against the ground, my teeth shattered, my nose split open, the vice grip on my hair pulled me backwards, then smashed me forwards.

A moment, a minute or a lifetime later, it came for me. Not sleep this time, but something similar. A caramel-thick blood-warm sensation enclosed me; as though floating on a breeze, all my pain began to dissolve. Separated sweetly from the agony, I decided it was my time to leave. Drifting away in pure peace and quiet, supple, figureless, distilled down, I started towards the dappled sunlight behind my closed eyes. As I slipped away, a whisper filled the void, echoing around me as though I was within the sound itself. *Please – don't go*, the voice said. *Please.*

So, just like a girl waiting patiently on the sidelines for her turn to join in the jump rope, when the rhythm of my convulsing body allowed, I slotted back into the game.

Later, I would come to know that this voice was Mum's voice, although she has no recollection of explicitly saying those words, but I suppose when a person is that close to death, the inexplicable is inevitable.

After the crash, I was ambulanced to the closest hospital and rushed into intensive care. For two days, I lay in critical condition, spinning in and out of consciousness, unaware of my surroundings or my body, my attention fixed only on the searing pain in my face, which had been split in half. My skull was fractured, my eye socket smashed, my jaw broken, my nose crushed. A surgeon would find fragments of it in my lungs. I had inhaled it.

When I was lucid, I was assured that none of my passengers were injured. Celia had suffered a minor head injury and was brought in to see me using a wheelchair as a precaution, and in my confusion, I panicked that I had disabled her, and I had a seizure. After that, they didn't bring the others in, or if they did, I have no memory of it.

I had no idea where I was, but I knew my family was orbiting around me constantly, because I never woke up alone. Their presence pulled me back like smelling salts. I woke to see Mum sleeping fully-dressed on the floor next to my hospital bed, her arm outstretched as though we had fallen asleep holding hands, and I wondered miserably what trouble I had caused her this time.

The hospital in Scotland was not equipped to deal with my injuries, so three days after the crash, I was flown to London for specialist treatment at the Royal National Orthopaedic Hospital. On arrival, my spine was immediately fixed with two eight-inch metal rods and eight two-inch screws, an eight-hour operation, after which my body was taken to recovery, where I lay almost lifeless, sucking on an oxygen mask.

Whatever was happening to my body seemed peripheral to the discomfort in my face, however; I couldn't breathe properly, my nose felt as though it had been packed with concrete, and no matter how hard I tried to fill my lungs with air, I simply couldn't.

My family had travelled south separately to me and arrived at the hospital the day after, hopeful the spinal fusion had improved my chances of survival, only to be told that my lungs were filling with fluid and they should prepare themselves for the worst. It had been five days since the crash, my body was failing. I began to die.

But as I drifted away, a man who was visiting another patient in the bed opposite saw my mum standing next to my bed holding up an X-ray of my spine and another of my face, and introduced himself to her. The man was called Peter Ayliffe, and he happened to be an expert in maxillofacial surgery, with specific interest in the reconstruction of the face and jaw. At first Mum didn't understand how he had come to be there, the coincidence frightened her. But when Peter looked at my X-rays and told Mum that he could help me, she decided to put her trust in synchronicity. My face would need to be reconstructed, he explained, so that I could breathe, but I would have to be transferred to a different hospital, where he worked. The doctors told my parents that I had only *just* survived the flight south, any further travel might kill me, but there was no other choice.

I regained consciousness around the same time as Mum made a decision about what to do. 'Take her and fix her,' she said, in that commanding tone I recognised and knew could only be her. She was looking at Peter as though he was the light at the end of a tunnel. He nodded back at her. I didn't understand what they were talking about, but I put my trust in him because Mum had.

He walked over to me and leant over, lifting up an oxygen mask I didn't even know was on my face, and he took a moment to smile at me as he assessed me.

'Hi, Sophie. I'm Peter Ayliffe and I am going to help you.' He winked at me kindly and I tried to wink hello, but even that hurt. Peter scanned my injuries and then said to my mum, 'I would like to try to repair the damage so that she looks as much like herself as possible. Do you happen to have any recent photos of Sophie?'

Mum yelped. She reached for her handbag and tipped everything out on to the floor.

'Peter, *look*, look what I have ... I don't believe it; we only took these a few days ago. Here she is,' Mum cried as she found the packet of freshly developed photos. She pointed at my face, proof that I'd once existed.

'Look, here she is—' Mum's voice broke. 'That was my girl ... '

*

Two days later, I woke up to find none of my family around me. Frightened, I waited a moment, scanning around with my one working eye. No one came. Lying on my back, unable to move, I tried to call for someone to be with me. My jaw wouldn't move, I tried to wiggle it, it didn't move, and still no one came. I tried to force my tongue through my teeth but I couldn't prise them apart. I began to panic. I moaned louder, a despairing sorrowful noise unlike any I'd heard myself make before.

Instead of my family, two men arrived at my hospital bed and without a word disconnected my body from the multiple outlets I was plugged into and started to move me. My stomach lurched, and every wound on my face began to throb in a pulsating chorus. As the men moving my bed gathered pace towards the door, my head erupted in a silent cacophony of pain. I began to retch but the men didn't stop. My bed kept rolling. I was riding the rollercoaster alone, screaming on the inside. I blacked out.

When I woke up, the men were attaching the various wires that connected my chest into a set of machines. I peeked through one eye as blood filled my mouth, the gagging had ripped open my gums.

'Thank you, porters,' said a bubbly nurse. 'The next one is ready for you to take down to theatre. He's in the bay next door.'

The two men left my side and, in their place, stood a stout thirty-something white man with a skinhead, rosy cheeks and warm, smiling hazelnut-brown eyes.

'Hello, darling, my name is Gary. I will be your nurse from now on. How are you? Sweetheart, if I'm honest, you don't look too good. In case you don't know, you have just had reconstructive surgery on your face; your nose has been rebuilt and your jaw has been wired, petal.' *That's why I couldn't open it*, I thought, panic rising again, feeling claustrophobic inside my own face. Gary continued, 'Your eye socket has also been repaired and bandaged. Your surgeon Mr Ayliffe told me you very nearly lost it, poor sausage. You have been brought back to the Royal National Orthopaedic Hospital, which is where you had your spinal fusion, okay? Now, if you had to rate your pain between one and ten, with ten being the worst, what are you?'

Wondering what a spinal fusion meant, I unclenched my two hands.

'Oh blimey, lovey, that many fingers, eh? Let me get the morphine hooked up so we can get that number down to a single figure, shall we?'

Gary twirled around and began expertly connecting wires and cables, all the while humming a calm low murmur to himself. The light in the room softened and a gentle breeze wafted over my body.

'Here. Take this and promise me that whenever you start to feel sore, you press this button. The clicker won't work immediately, but what this will do is release more morphine straight into your veins so that you can keep the pain away. It's a godsend, I tell ya!'

Gary placed a small grey clicker into my palm. I pressed it several times.

'Look at those puppy eyes.' Gary giggled and cleared some of the blood off my chin. He spoke to me as though I was a baby, but I didn't mind. In fact, I didn't want him to stop talking to me. I didn't know where I was or where my family was and he was so chirpy and calming, I felt safe with him. Taking a little breather, Gary looked closer at my face. As if reading my mind he said, 'Your family have gone home for the day, but I met your mum yesterday, and I'm arranging a room for her in the nurses' quarters, so she can be closer to you. She'll be back tomorrow first thing. Don't worry, darling, I will look after you in the meantime. Now, let me see inside your mouth, is It okay if I, can I just . . . ?'

Gary gently curled my top lip up and grimaced. 'Oh, you poor love. Let me get you some water to rinse away all the blood. Are you feeling nauseous as well?'

I nodded.

'Right, I'll get you some anti-nausea injections immediately. You lie still and try to relax. You are here now, and you don't need to move again. This is the Spinal Rehabilitation Unit, your home for, well, for as long as it takes . . .'

Gary spun round and trotted out the door.

Takes to what? I thought, but before that terrifying train of thought carried me somewhere I didn't want to go yet, the morphine arrived in my bloodstream and underneath the quiet breeze, I drifted away.

The Spinal Unit

A week later, I lay looking at the clock on the wall.
Quarter past three.

I'd seen every angle those hands could be at, every possible moment of every possible minute of every possible hour.

Sixteen minutes past three.

I sucked in some saliva. It tasted foul and smelt like nothing I had smelt before, but I'd got used to it. In fact, this stomach-churning stench had claimed everything around me – the air, my body, people, food, not that there was much food, but whatever there was, it reeked of this smell.

Fluid ran out of my nose, trickling down to my painfully cracked lips. I winced. Tears leaked out from under the bandage, and as I'd done with every tear that had leaked down my face since the morning, I tried to trace the feel of it, but my face was numb and it was only when it reached my cracked lips and the salt stung, that I felt it.

Another tear fell. The process started all over again.

Seventeen minutes past three.

Through my left eye I took in my surroundings. The hospital room was small and light, with a door on my left that led to what I thought might be a garden. On my right was a glass window that looked over the spinal unit, and beside that a door that, as yet, I hadn't seen closed. Blinds were drawn against the doors so that my room stayed private, and for all the uncertainty and unfamiliarity, there was a sense of sanctity in the space.

Some cards had been pinned to a board opposite my bed and from where I lay, I could just make out the writing. None of them, I noticed, said 'get well soon'; 'condolences', I thought, were for dead people?

Someone had pinned up a photograph: Tom and I play-fighting in the sunshine. Mum must have got the disposable camera developed. The photos might only have been taken just over a fortnight ago, but it felt like a distant memory. What did the laughing girl in that photo do to me?

I squeezed on the morphine clicker, but it didn't stop the image of her from stinging.

I wished someone would take it down.

I looked back at the clock.

Eighteen minutes past three.

I was beginning to land from wherever my mind had been, back into my body, but it didn't feel like a body. Only a face. Under the morphine, the pulsating pain was lessening, or at least I could isolate and identify what exactly was hurting, what was itching, what might be bleeding or what was throbbing. Stitches pinched and stung when I twitched.

I didn't have any idea what my face looked like but it felt altered. Nobody had offered me a mirror – I took that as a hint. Besides, any time someone came into my room and looked at me, I could tell from their reactions it would be best for me to wait before I looked for myself.

Looking at my family was distressing enough. Dad's eyes were so swollen he looked as though he was crying even when he had stopped. Gone were the blue-grey twinkly eyes and boyish blond wispy hair of the Dad I remembered. He had aged

so drastically he was almost unrecognisable. The man who followed Mum into my room each day had greasy unwashed hair
and the pallid complexion of someone who had forgotten how
to sleep. He looked vulnerable, and that made me want to look
away. I knew that hospitals scared him, but I had never seen
that fear actualised before. I watched him as the nurses cared
for me and could tell the hierarchy confused him: which nurse
did what and which doctor was who? He hung back and kept
quiet. If he did ask any questions they were stuttered and confused. I longed to hug him and tell him he could go home. My
brother stood by his side, pinching at the skin on his hands like
he used to when he was little, when I would get us in trouble.
The skin looked raw.

The two of them looked to Mum to translate to us all what
was happening.

Mum stood guarding my bed as though she were one of her
working dogs, growling at anyone who came close. She had a
pad of paper and a pen, and every time a new face approached
me, Mum asked for their name and role, and wrote it down as
though to warn them that whatever they did to this particular
patient, in this specific room, they would be held accountable.
As though there was an unspoken understanding of how traumatised mothers behave, no one refused her; they knew she was
just trying to keep me safe.

'I'm not taking any fucking risks,' she barked. 'I've done this
job. I *know* how tired people get. I know the mistakes that get
made ... That's not happening, not on my watch.'

My tortured mother appeared to me like a sad clown, her eyes
dead below her make-up and her mouth forced upwards into
a clenched smile as though the corners of her rictus grin were
trying to hold her whole body up.

Thankfully, when Mum brought Sara in with her, the mood
was lighter. Although Sara had always been like a mother to me,

the fact that she wasn't was immediately evident; she wasn't as devastated as Mum, she was one step removed, not in the same boat, but in the same storm, so to speak, and this positioned her perfectly to support us all. When she stood beside Mum, she seemed almost to hoick her up, as though Mum's legs were seconds away from collapsing under her from tiredness. I wondered if she had eaten anything other than cigarettes. The familiar smell of her perfume curdled with smoke and added to my perpetual state of nausea.

I'd never had to read my family before; if I needed to know something about how they were feeling or what they were thinking I'd ask, or they would tell me. But I was realising that, in this new reality, I would have to understand the things that people *weren't* saying to me; the secondary conversation that was happening underneath – the one without words – was where the truth lay.

So when Mum checked over my face each morning, studying every cut and bruise for signs of progress or deterioration, I studied her face right back. She hovered over my eye and looked pleased; over my nose she twitched a little; she peeled back a lip and flinched; then she pulled in her breath, closed her eyes, took a moment for a thought, and opened them and smiled at me. But the smile wasn't honest. I didn't believe it for a second. I had been keeping silent to minimise the pain, and for self-preservation; if one word came out then so too might some questions and I was determined to stay as ignorant as possible about what had happened to me. The pain in my face was all I wanted to think about, not the terrifying nothingness of the rest of me. But Mum's bravery killed me.

'I'm so sorry, Mum . . .' I whispered.

She jumped in fright, and as her guard went down, for the first time in my life I saw her not as my mum but as a person. A person in shock. A woman heartbroken. A mother in ruins.

I realised then, given her nursing background, that she would have known exactly what was happening to me and she must have felt so alone in the face of the truth.

'Please don't apologise to me, Sophie. There is nothing to be sorry about, it was an *accident* and everyone else is fine. You ... everything is going to, everything, will, it's all going to be okay ... *okay* ... '

She was looking despondently at the space between us and the words seemed to fall from her mouth, heavily laden with doubt. Nothing had ever frightened me more than hearing such a distinct lack of conviction from my mother.

I saved my energy and returned to silence because if I knew anything about her, I knew she wouldn't be wasting her time trying to make sense of whatever had happened, she would be keeping busy trying to find ways to help me. It would be best to save the apologies for another time, when she might hear them. (I'm sorry, Mum.)

Thankfully, most of the time, the fuzzy cushion of morphine kept me separated from both the pain and the reality and let the goings-on around me feel dreamlike.

One morning I lay snoozing, lusciously tripping out, when a cleaner crept into my room to mop and tidy. As he was so stealthy it was his mop not him that stirred me, as it swished water across the floor. I caught his eye and he smiled directly at me.

Reluctant to try to talk through my wired jaw, I smiled back and winked, and without a word he held my smile, as he continued mopping. He'd put his radio on my tray table. He was almost dancing as he moved. Seeing me look towards it, he gestured to ask me if I wanted him to turn up the volume. I nodded.

As the music reached me, I had to stop myself from crying out. His smile grew into a wide knowing beam. The song was so significant, I snuffed with laughter, at the lyrics and because this was the first bit of music I'd heard since the party back before this had happened. 'What a Wonderful World' by Louis Armstrong.

As the cleaner danced around the room, he pulled back the blinds into the garden. Behind him, a low slow strobe light of sunshine caught my eye and I remembered that it was still summer out there. The room turned a warm yellow. All of a sudden it felt like hope had returned.

This was the first track I'd played in my car after I passed my driving test, and I'd named my first car, a clapped-out rusty red Peugeot 106, Louis. The day I got Louis, Ellie and I had driven straight to Halfords and bought some fluffy pink dice for the rear-view mirror and a fake exhaust to make him look more beastly on the road. We fancied ourselves boy racers, pushing Louis to his limits on the country roads around our school. At the thought of us speeding through the countryside, with the windows down and some trance music pounding, even in my stillness, I felt a rush. *It* is *a beautiful world*, and the summer was out there; Ellie – and all the people I loved – were out there, and one day, I would be out there again too.

Whatever had happened to bring me to a spinal unit would surely be fixed soon.

Run, girl, run

By the end of my first week at the spinal unit, I started to know the routine of the day.

Every morning at around five, the lights would flicker through the ward, waking those who, like me, lay lightly on the surface of sleep. A team of nurses would then rouse those still deep asleep, safe in the sanctuary of their own minds, where most of us longed to remain, without pain or suffering.

I had been put in a room by myself, but through my door I could hear other patients hanging on to their pillows for dear life, moans and cries echoing around the ward. Undeterred and cheerful, the nurses would get to work on our bodies, rolling up the covers as our eyes peeled open and, fussing and chatting, start on our morning routines. I'd stay quiet and play a guessing game with my senses, my knuckles white on the morphine clicker.

I'd hear a count of three and then I would be twisted over to one side. Then water and the sounds of washing and the smell of soap. One, two, three, back to the centre again. I tried to feel for where their hands were, but there was no sensation, nothing registering. Not even numbness. And then, the nurse's cold hands and the hints of a sponge around the top of my back. The soapy warm rubs gently worked their way towards my neck, wiping away the sweat, pus, dribble and blood deposited there by my face. My face they didn't touch. I vibrated ever so slightly as my body was patted dry.

As the nurses moved around my body, they used a word that I couldn't understand and one morning, my curiosity getting the better of me, I croaked up at them through my wired jaw.

'Hello,' I said politely, 'peass . . . ' And both nurses gave a little yelp. I hadn't got the hang of speaking through the wired jaw and the word 'please' came out like a loose fart. I gulped and sucked in some straying saliva. 'I keep hearing you talk about "ssuuubss", I'd like to know what ish meansss . . . peass?'

'Oh, sweetheart, you mean "sups". Short for suppositories. Suppositories.' She repeated the world slowly like I wasn't really all there. 'We insert them into your rectum to stimulate your bowels. You'll learn all about this in due course so don't worry. You see, you aren't able to control your bowels any more, darling, so we are managing them for you.'

What the fuck did she just say? Surely this woman was mistaken.

I tried to turn around to challenge her, but she had me pinned on one side. It was then I noticed a large bag of urine hanging over the side of my bed. I felt a cold wave rush over my face, washing away any expression I may have had. I followed the tube from the bag, tracking it all the way until it disappeared beneath my hospital gown. It dawned on me that I hadn't had a wee for as long as I could remember. Come to think of it, the last time I had been in a toilet was at the party, posing in that mirror.

Uninvited, questions forced their way out of my darkest fears: *Where had the nurses been washing me? Where did the tube of urine go?* I didn't have time to voice the questions before my weight shifted once again, as the nurses – one, two, three – moved me around further, before returning me on to my back where they left me.

'Right, lovey,' one of them said, smiling at me, 'I have put the sups in your rectum, they will get to work, and I will be back in about half an hour to manually evacuate your bowels.'

And with that they moved on.

A part of my mind seemed instinctively tuned in to the lack of communication from my lower limbs, but another part, still deeply in denial, attempted then to test the line of communication. I tried to move and then feel my body, but each time there was no feedback. The line was dead.

Where was that tube running to?

I could feel my arms and hands, and I twitched them to check; I could move them. Whatever was stopping me from controlling the rest of me would be fixed soon, I thought again. *Surely.* Everything else was mending. The pain in my face was lessening every day. Don't panic. *Don't shit the bed* . . . Suddenly that expression took on a whole new meaning. And it was not fucking funny.

I brought a hand up to my face, appreciating the simplicity of this action for the first time in my life. There were tan lines across my fingers where my rings had been removed. Even in the white clinical depths of this despair, I still carried the suntan from my previous life. Memories of travelling in the summer felt fresh on my fingertips.

From inside this room, behind this proverbial sliding door, I wondered where *she* was, the other me. The one in the photo. I looked at her on the wall. Had she gone through a different door, taken the blue pill and perhaps gone into the life I had dreamed for her? I hoped so. I hoped she was free and running far away from whatever was happening here with her chunky legs and freshly shaven pussy, with her life – and her bowels – under her control.

Lightly as a feather I reached up to my face; nervously my index finger found and followed thick stitches from my lip all the way up to my forehead. My left eye lay out of reach beneath a bandage so I went higher, into my hairline, but it was matted and thick and impenetrable. My fingernails scratched my scalp, there was dirt and what appeared to be dried blood; I tried to smell it, but the smell of my new nose prevailed. I went carefully back in and found stitches in my scalp. I tracked them through my hairline down towards my right ear. I flicked at a protruding stitch, and the wound it held together stung.

What had I done to myself?

The nurses returned and through the one eye that I could see through, I watched as they arranged themselves around my body.

'Now, lovey, we are going to turn you back on to your side and empty your bowels.'

Was that other me dancing on a tabletop in a club somewhere? My thoughts strayed as the women counted down from three and turned me over. *Was she running in the woods with her naughty mates?* I felt the bed rock and my body move within it. The nurses chatted to one another about their lousy shift hours. *Maybe she was on a flight, off on an adventure?* A smell reached my nose and filtered past the clots of dried blood. The stench of shit filled the air. I gagged painfully. *Or perhaps she was in bed with Rory, being licked on that shaven haven?*

'There we go, lovey. You seem constipated so best up your water intake.'

I didn't reply.

The line to my body remained dead.

Question Time

At the start of the second week I was lying watching the second hand of the clock, when I heard the familiar clop of Mum's boots arriving on the ward: 8 a.m. on the dot.

'Morning, Phie Phie.' She kissed me carefully, checking every bruise and stitch for progress as usual. Satisfied, she walked over to the sink and filled a small plastic cup with water before hunting down my toothbrush and a straw.

'Here you go, darling. Try to clean your teeth. It will make you feel a little more human. Would you like an Ensure or shall I crush up a banana for you for breakfast?' Ensure, a smoothie drink packed with thousands of calories, had been keeping me alive, alongside intravenous steroids. The synthetic taste had curdled with the putrid smell of newness and made me want to throw up, but Gary had told me I needed to gain weight. I didn't have much of an appetite; shitting in a bag will do that to you.

I nodded as Mum passed me the cup and I began to ease the toothbrush between my chapped lips in an attempt to freshen the space between the metal clamps inside. But I stopped.

'Mum, can I have a mirror today?' I croaked.

'Of course you can, sweetheart, but ...' Mum reached into her bag. 'Are you sure you're ready?'

I wasn't but I nodded. Mum passed me a mirror and planted a kiss on my forehead. 'I love you, Phie.'

'Love you too. Can I be alone, Mum?'

'Of course, I'll go and get you the smoothie *and* the banana.' Mum was so hesitant to leave me alone, she walked backwards out of the door. I waited till she was gone then brought the mirror to my face. I almost stopped breathing. Black stitches ran haphazardly down the centre of my face, and where once was a long, smooth nose, now was a violently misshapen mountain-range of cartilage. The bruises under my eyes were deep purple, black in parts. My right eye was bandaged but I could see red stains on the white, evidence of the damage underneath. But it wasn't the battered shapes or vivid bruises or chaotic stitches that took my breath away; it was that the face in the mirror looked vacantly back at me. She looked exactly how I felt: scared and dazed. She looked traumatised. We blinked. The photo of me on the wall caught my eye. I looked back between it and my reflection. A single tear escaped from under the bandage.

Feebly, I brought my toothbrush to my mouth, but I was so dumbstruck, I slipped, the toothbrush cutting into my gum, and I spluttered out the white froth. I tried to clean it up, but a wire in my arm got tangled up and I yanked it by mistake, pulling my skin apart. I cried out.

To distract my mind from the pain and any ensuing nausea, I tried to calm myself, but my worried mind wandered to the one place I didn't want it to.

What had happened that night? Where was Jack? Where was Rory? Where were my friends? And the worst and loudest concern of all: what had I done to my body?

Unable to sit upright, I held the mirror up and used it to look down to my body, as though searching for a bomb. I saw my toes at the end of the bed and tried to wiggle them but they didn't move. I wiggled the mirror instead, trying not to scream.

The morphine hit my empty stomach and turned my skin a pale shade of green. I threw the mirror out of my reach.

'Right, here we are—' Mum had returned with breakfast. 'Oh darling, what's wrong?'

Tears patted down to my pillow, but I stopped them instantly. She looked so tired I didn't have the heart to burden her with my worries. Plus, I told myself angrily, I was eighteen, her mothering duties were meant to be over. These tears were my bitter pills to swallow, not hers. After all of the suffering I had caused her in my childhood, whatever I had done to myself was *my* punishment, I *deserved* this not her, and I should be carrying my pain alone, that's what adults are supposed to do.

'It's nothing, Mum,' I lisped through my teeth, clearing my throat as gently as I could.

'Okay, Phie, I have to tighten the bands on your jaw today. Sorry, but it's going to hurt.' Mum reached into one of the bedside cupboards for a pair of tweezers, placing the breakfast drink in my hand as she passed. I had never been her patient before. Gloves on, she gently prised my mouth apart and, after dabbing away the toothpaste I'd trailed down my chin, she used the tweezers to grip on to the first of fifteen small rubber bands that were stretched over what looked much like braces screwed into my gum line, connecting the upper and lower jaws. 'Do you want to watch in the mirror?'

I nodded and she handed me the mirror again. I put down my breakfast drink and held the mirror back up to my face. As slowly as she could she unhooked the lower part of the band, then twisted it and reattached it, tightening the braces so my jaw was more firmly closed. Twist, clench, twist.

It was a good thing I couldn't open my mouth, otherwise I'd have yelled.

Blood trickled out from my gum.

As she moved on to the next, my knuckles blanched.

'Fourteen more to go.' Loudly and deliberately, Mum relaxed the rhythm of her breath, encouraging me to relax as best as she could.

'Only a few more weeks till these come off. Only a few more weeks ...'

Half an hour later, Mum wrapped up the first of her morning's jobs with a kiss on my forehead.

'There we go. That wasn't *too* bad now, was it?' Mum's nursing manner relaxed me.

'Morning, princess. Is your mum in yet? Oh, hi, Carol!' Gary and Mum exchanged greetings like they were old friends. 'How's your face today then, Sophie? Better! Much better! I see your mum has done your bands. How's the eye? Oooh ... ouch. Looks sore. And what about your back?' Gary vigorously turned me to inspect my back. I moaned as pain like red-hot pokers jutted in my back and I felt a sharp crack in my arm. 'Oh sorry, darling, I forgot about your collarbone.'

My collarbone? 'Huh?' I pressed down harder on the morphine tap.

'You snapped your clavicle, so we haven't been turning you on that side. I *totally* forgot, sorry. In other news, though, the stitches in your back seem to be healing well.'

'Gary ...' The time had come to ask someone. 'I don't seem to be able to, er, control my body any more.' The freshly tightened wiring was causing my mouth to throb again. I took a deep breath through my clenched jaw. 'What happened to my back? What happened to *me*?'

Gary paused. Mum had heard my question, so she stepped forward and held my hand.

'Darling, your back was cut open so that metal rods could be placed around your spine to protect it and stop any further damage from happening.'

'Okay.' I sucked in more saliva. 'But *why*?'

'You crashed the car you were driving and, in the crash . . . ' Gary cleared his throat and looked at Mum. In the pause I had a flashback. I was upside down in a field, I could taste mud. *Was I upside down with my cunt exposed?* Someone was talking to me, reassuring me . . . The memory stopped there. Mum took over from Gary.

'Darling, they suspect the vertebrae of your spine were twisted, because your spinal cord has been damaged . . . ' I tried to piece bits together: my gut instinct, the comments from the nurses, the name of the ward, the unnerving abyss below me, the inability to move. I waited, frozen, with my broken heart in my broken mouth, to hear Mum's words out loud.

'Phie, you've had a spinal cord injury. You're paralysed and . . . ' She didn't fake a smile or try to hold back. 'You won't ever walk again.'

When they left me some unknown time later, my eyes found the hands of the clock once again, and for a while, I followed the second hand. The sound of the sharp definitive ticks grew louder in my consciousness and I let the tapping take over so that I would not have to try to make sense of what I had just heard. Tick, tick, tick.

Never walk again. Never walk again. *I matched the words with the rhythm of time. Can I stop the clock? Can I go back?*

I tried to think back, to retrace my steps, the last steps of my life.

Before I got into the car, I was walking beside Rory. My black dress skimmed my tanned knees, my legs had got used to the heels and my hips swayed casually. We had come out of the party – I played back the evening in my mind as though rewinding a video. I saw myself dancing, my blonde hair flicked around me and my arms raised in the air. Sweat trickled down my back. Before that, I was with Jack. We were arguing about ending things.

I was distracted.

I had no idea I was on the edge of a cliff, with a blindfold on, about to fall off . . .

Tick, tick, tick.

Never. Walk. Again.

I slept, but once again, the figure by the car waited for me, and this time, he had a face.

The next day, Gary stood beside my bed, one tattooed hand resting on my arm, the other around Mum, who had on a fresh shirt and, I noticed, clean hair. Opposite them, two women, one wearing a green uniform and one in blue, both of whom I'd never seen before but I instinctively liked. Firstly, because one of them sauntered into my room with her hands in her pockets and nodded hello at me as casually as if we were meeting in the pub for a pint and I needed that type of energy, and secondly because the other, the smaller of the two, had gone straight up to Mum and hugged her as though this were the most natural and appropriate way to greet a perfect stranger.

Whatever their jobs, they looked the sort to be able to salvage someone like me from the wreckage.

The taller one spoke first. 'Hello, Sophie, my name is Emma and I'll be your occupational therapist. This is Debbie, your physio.' The smaller woman gave me a friendly nod and picked up a folder with my name on it from the end of the bed. Emma continued. 'It's been three weeks since you sustained your spinal cord injury, and while you've been in recovery, we've been taking "prick" tests to assess the severity of your paralysis and we can confirm that you have a spinal cord injury at the vertebra six of the thoracic part of the spine, and our tests would indicate that below the level of this injury you have what we call complete paralysis—'

'A "complete" injury,' Gary clarified, 'differs from the more commonly sustained "incomplete" injuries, in which a person may regain some movement or feeling after spinal injury, especially with extra physiotherapy or other therapies—'

'Basically, what this means, Soph, is that as a thoracic six complete paraplegic, you'll have *no* movement and *no* sensation below the level of your breasts.'

Something about Emma's straight-talking suited me. No fluff or bullshit, just the facts. Nevertheless, I looked at Mum to try to help me understand how to respond to what I'd been told. She used to joke to Dad, 'if I want your opinion, I'll give it to you', and this was what I wanted.

But Mum let Emma continue.

'With a *complete* spinal cord injury, of your level, we expect you to live an independent and full life, and it's our job to help that happen, to help you get there. But I want you to know now it's best not to expect or hope for any change in your condition. With a complete level, it's unlikely that you will recover any feeling or sensation again.'

'Mum?' I needed to hear it from her.

'No, darling . . . apparently, not ever.'

I didn't know how to respond. I didn't know what thoracic meant. In those lessons when I was supposed to be learning about how bodies work, I had been too busy reading Jilly Cooper novels under my desk, but I didn't want to admit my ignorance. Frightened doesn't come close to describing how I felt, neither does shocked. My brain simply wasn't able to compute it all.

But, it occurred to me, no one was actually asking me how I felt, nor was anyone crying or breaking down at that moment. No matter how terminal and unchangeable or life-changing it all was, what I was *not* being told was that my life was over. Emma seemed so relaxed and laid-back, we may as well have been in the pub discussing what to drink next, and this soothed me enormously.

'What happens now,' Emma continued, 'is that you'll begin your rehabilitation, which will be overseen by myself, Debbie, Gary and your spinal consultant. There's a process, and we'll take you step by step—' I snorted in disagreement and to my surprise Emma laughed, rolling her eyes to admit her mistake. 'Oh, you know what I mean, not step by step – we will take you, bit by bit, through each process so that eventually you'll be able to leave here independently.'

Laughter in the presence of such trauma felt as helpful as any drug I had been given so far. I smiled at Emma, flashing the metalwork in my mouth like a child with braces.

'Sophie, darling,' Debbie now took over. 'We know this will feel overwhelming for you and you'll have a ton of questions. That's what we – and Gary, of course – are here for. Okay? We have a folder here that we'll leave with you with information about spinal cord injury. Each section has a test at the end and once you've completed them all, we'll know that you're almost ready to go home.'

Debbie handed me a plastic folder. I opened it and held it above my face. There were sections running down the spine that read, 'Bladder', 'Bowel Management', 'Skin', 'Autonomic Dysreflexia', 'The Respiratory System', 'Sexual Function'. I slapped it shut, lay it on my stomach and looked at the two women.

'How long will it take?' I spoke as clearly as I could.

'How long will what take?'

'Till I can get my life back again?'

'Well . . . ' Emma said. 'That all depends on what you want your life to be.'

I thanked her for her honesty with a decisive nod, yet remained uncertain.

'You want some water, princess?' Gary said, and I noticed he had been holding Mum's hand to support her. He let her go and walked over to the sink. This nickname for me was far from accurate, no princess would look or feel (or smell) as awful as I did in that moment, but I let it go because while I may not have been anything like a *princess*, it felt hopeful, like a label to aim for. *Paraplegic*, on the other hand, did not. I had no idea what that label embodied.

Emma told me she'd be back in the morning for our first session and Debbie gave the folder on my stomach a quick tap. 'Whenever you're ready, Sophie; there is no rush. Your face needs to mend a little more before we *really* get started, so take your time?'

Gary handed me some water, gave Mum a consoling squeeze, scooped up the women and off they went. For the first time, he closed the door behind him.

Mum and I looked at each other, but we didn't speak. We just locked eyes and stayed still. But in the secondary conversation – the one we didn't have out loud, the one that carried from her soul to mine, like an imaginary placenta – I found all that I needed to hear.

Manual of Doom

The folder was marked with the letters SCI in black marker pen, and underneath, in bold capital letters, the words 'Spinal Cord Injury'.

After I had left school I had made a point of burning all of my folders. Looking at this new one, on a topic no one would ever want to take, I sighed. I had tasted freedom for two months, or eight weeks, or fifty-six whole days, and here I was, back being schooled again. But if learning the content would help me get a semblance of a life back, then so be it, I would study it and obey it, to the letter. If ever there was a time to be an A student, it was now, and if I completed the folder quickly, maybe I would be able to leave hospital sooner. I looked at the first page.

'Spinal Injury'. Bracing myself, I read on. 'The spine consists of a chain of bones called vertebrae, which provides support for our whole body, linking head, shoulders, chest and pelvis. It is very strong to support the body weight (supple discs between the vertebrae absorb shock) and it is flexible, to allow turning and bending. Each section of the backbone is given a name and each vertebra is given a number.'

I looked for the thoracic six, right in the middle of the diagram.

'The spinal cord is within the spine, about as thick as a finger, and it attaches to the brain at the base of the skull and runs up and down the length of the back inside the backbone; it is made up of bundles of nerve fibres carrying messages from the brain to all parts of the body. There are three kinds of messages or signals which travel along the spinal cord; sensory, motor and reflexes.'

I looked at one of my fingers. The thickness of it seemed so insubstantial, how could damage to something so small be so catastrophic? I skipped ahead to the section about 'Complete Injuries'.

'With a complete spinal injury there will not be any feeling or movement below the level of injury. A complete spinal cord injury changes the control of all the functions of the nervous system.'

According to the manual I would no longer be able to feel hot or cold touch, nor pain nor pressure.

I fact-checked this information, closing my eyes to try to test the line, but again, nothing. What about the sun on my skin? Or water? What about mud in my toes? Or *stubbing* my toe? What about waxing my legs or someone sitting on my lap? I tried to control the questions from spiralling out of control.

The manual went on to explain that 'after the spinal cord injury, messages below the level of the injury are unable to get past the damage in the spinal cord; no feeling or sensory messages would come back up to the brain either. Bowel, bladder and sexual function may also change after a spinal cord injury. There may also be changes in breathing, temperature control, heart rate and blood pressure.' It explained each injury is like a fingerprint, unique to the person to whom the injury happens. Car crashes, knife wounds, cliff jumps, rugby scrums, horse riding, domestic violence, cancer tumours are all known causes of spinal injury and so complex is the recovery that the treatment must be highly specialised, which is why, according to what I was reading, I was so fortunate to have a bed at one of the UK's leading spinal hospitals The Royal National Orthopaedic Hospital in Stanmore, north London.

I read that I was also fortunate to have sustained my injury in 2003. In the past, if a person were to suffer a spinal injury, their chance of survival was poor. Until Professor Guttmann, an exiled Jewish surgeon from Nazi Germany, devised a rehabilitation programme in 1944, most of those who sustained a spinal injury would have fallen victim to a urinary tract infection or pressure sore and died, but Guttmann found ways to keep patients alive and enabled them to rebuild their lives. His rehabilitation programme included enabling his patients to play sports, to keep them motivated and fit. It worked so well that in time other hospitals followed his lead and soon an army of paraplegics and quadriplegics from around the country was formed. Guttmann brought them together to compete against one another in sport, primarily archery, and this competition eventually turned into what is now called the Paralympic Games.

Numbly, I flicked ahead to the first section marked 'Bladder'.

A clinical diagram of the urinary system marking out where the urethra, bladder and kidneys were was printed on the page, and below it another simplified summary of how this most natural bodily function had been impacted. 'After a spinal injury, the bladder will no longer work as it did before the injury.' I skimmed ahead, plucking out details that related to my specific injury, 'the urge to empty the bladder will not be felt'.

My eyes glazed over and, unable to focus on the words, I looked instead to the drawings: a cross-section of a bladder, with what looked like a clear plastic straw inserted into it through the urethra; then below that a photograph of a human stomach with a tube inserted into the skin; and below that an image of a penis with a condom over it, filled with urine. It was nightmarish.

I moved on to the next section: 'Skin'. The manual explained I could no longer feel my lower body from the chest down so I would have to be constantly vigilant, checking the temperature of anything that could cause my stomach or legs to get too cold or hot. My hypothalamus could no longer communicate with my brain, so, below my level of injury, I would no longer sweat either, and no longer be able to regulate my body temperature. I could easily become a victim of overheating or freezing.

The word 'victim' jumped out at me. I had never known the strength of the repulsion it triggered in me before because I had never been considered one. Horrified, I read on. 'If there is no feeling below the injury level, no warning signals will tell you when you have hurt yourself . . . after spinal cord injury, messages or signals are not able to get to the brain to tell you when to move . . . sitting or lying too long cuts off the blood flow in the skin . . . blood flow to the skin keeps it alive and healthy; if the skin does not get blood, it will die . . . with a complete spinal cord injury, you will not sweat or shiver below the level of injury. Loss of sweating below the level of injury can cause the skin to become dry and flaky, and sometimes crack . . . The most common cause of a skin sore is pressure. If the pressure is not relieved, it will get worse. The skin will become red, purple or black. Treatment at this stage may involve weeks or even months of bed-rest staying off the area . . . inspect your skin every morning and every night . . . Stick to your turn schedule at night—'

I'd had enough. Slamming the manual shut, I picked up the mirror.

I stared and stared at my reflection and prayed that the girl I once was would come to my rescue. If I couldn't have her body any more, I would *at least* need her strength to carry me out of here.

*

The following day, Emma came into my room and I asked her what she had planned.

'Well, today, *you* aren't going to be doing anything, but I am. I'm going to do some exercises on your legs so I just want you to try to relax. In fact, why don't you have a read of the folder?'

This wasn't so much of an invitation as an instruction. She passed it to me along with a pen. Emma didn't appear to be the needlessly chatty type, and as she went to work at the end of the bed, I dutifully reopened the manual of doom, trying not to think about every single sport I would now no longer be able to play.

It surprised me how thin and flimsy the folder was. Skimming through it, I would have expected there to be chapters on *all* of the questions I had, but it was broken down into just six sections.

Fresh from school, I knew exactly how to work through a workbook quickly. The material in the manual was a guide for living with spinal cord injury, and unlike mathematics or English, I *needed* to understand this subject. There was a curiosity in me I had never experienced before.

A few pages in, however, I had to stop.

Still unable to sit up or move, nurses had been routinely turning me every four hours, even through the night, and I had grown accustomed to being manhandled, but whatever Emma was doing to my legs was far more rigorous. She rocked me out of the sweaty groove I had moulded into my pillow.

'Don't mind me,' she said, as I looked at what she was doing. 'I'm just testing your reflexes and giving you some stretches.'

She had my leg in her arms and was flexing my ankle, and even though I'd just read that I couldn't feel or move my legs, I wasn't prepared for the vision of my own leg moving, without me having any control or sensation.

When the nurses had told me they were controlling my

bowels for me, it was almost possible to convince myself they were pretending, because I couldn't see what they were doing, but this was different. I could see, with my own eyes, and I couldn't fucking believe it, nor could I hide from it. I felt so disorientated, I thought I'd faint.

But yet again, Emma's professionalism and confidence reassured me. As I lay there watching her, I noticed that no matter how abnormal this situation, my body didn't upset or frighten her. She lifted my knees, flexed my hips and moved my legs, and while I knew this was her job and therefore entirely normal for her, that didn't lessen the impact it had on my understanding of my impairment. If she could be fearless of it, perhaps I could be too.

I picked up the manual of doom again and started to look through the pages for more images. An illustration of a tall thin woman alongside a young girl caught my eye. The woman was smiling, purposeful, dressed in the standardised uniform of a physio or carer, and below her, in a grey tracksuit and oversized T-shirt, sat the girl, expressionless and passive, in a wheelchair.

It wasn't the shape, size or colour of the chair, which, like the T-shirt, was too large for the girl, that made me stop. What bothered me was that her hands were folded in her lap. The girl was being pushed.

'Emma?' I said, but I wasn't sure what I wanted to ask.

Emma, who I noticed was not too dissimilar to the woman in the drawing, stopped what she was doing, carefully repositioned my limb, and leant over to check what I was looking at.

'Sophie,' she said, and there was a softness in her voice, 'you don't need to rush to that part yet; you aren't at that stage of your rehab.'

I flicked to the next page, trying to swipe away the image from my mind. But the passive hands in the girl's lap were difficult for me to unsee. Being pushed or depending on someone for help went against everything I knew. I'd taught myself how to tie my own shoelaces when I was a toddler, for crying out loud.

Emma turned the page back, looking more closely at the drawing she sensed had worried me, then she took the manual and placed it out of my reach.

'There are times when you will need to be pushed, Sophie, but most of the time you will be able to push yourself. You will have to learn how to manage yourself *by yourself*, and also learn how to ask for help when you need it. Try not to worry. You have so much to learn, I don't want you to overwhelm yourself. Once you're able to sit upright, you can think about learning to wash yourself and get dressed by yourself. After that I will teach you how to get in a wheelchair, and then, we'll go from there . . .'

Go where? I thought. *Where could anyone go in a wheelchair?*

'Okay, well, that's our session for today done. I'll be back at the same time tomorrow, and Debbie will be in in the morning. Is your mum still here?'

'No.' Mum had left quite suddenly earlier, looking excited, without much of an explanation.

'Okay, Soph, well done. See you tomorrow.'

With Emma's (and Mum's) steady presence gone, the room began to close in on me. They were telling me that a life was still possible but lying there alone in a body that I could not move, feel or control, I lost hold of that hope. The women in my life had shown me that I could be many things, but above all else, self-reliance, independence and strength mattered the most. My friends were further evidence that the wilder and freer the woman, the better. So, what exactly happens to a woman when she becomes *paralysed*? The lexicon of aspirational adjectives that I had been conditioned to attribute to the word 'woman' had never included *that* word. To be deaf, blind, paralysed, these were my most feared conditions of the human experience.

How could someone who had always been known as free-spirited, filthy, ravenous, rebellious, an incorrigible wild child, also be *paralysed*?

How could I be wild and trapped?

Baby Steps

Two weeks into rehabilitation, the time had come to start sitting me upright. Each morning, Gary raised the head of my hospital bed a little higher, inch by inch, until I was able to sit up without feeling dizzy or my blood pressure dropping. The movement may have been considered progress, but it felt pathetic to me, nevertheless. Everything that had once seemed easy and natural, in this new life, was a challenge. The only time I had needed help sitting up before was when I was drunk, I thought back longingly. The word 'paralytic' suddenly took on a whole new meaning.

After a couple of days, Gary eventually got me sitting.

Having been lying horizontally for so long, unable to see my lower body properly, I was almost able to forget it was there – out of sight, out of mind. But, as I sat up, resting against the back of the bed for balance, there they were – my legs. Still attached, still part of me, stretched out below me. Despite how it felt, my body looked entirely whole.

Gary saw me staring.

'You okay, princess?'

'Gary, can I wash myself today? Am I strong enough?'

'If you mean physically, yes, I think you are.' He gathered around me the gloves, wipes, pads, water, soap and towels. Still early in the morning, my bowels had been done already by the nurses. Mum was yet to arrive. The atmosphere in the ward was one of general busyness as other patients were being seen to.

As he closed the blinds he reminded me, 'If you are going to wash your face, just be careful around your eye.' Gary handed me my mirror with a proud look on his face, and left me alone with myself. I had no idea where to even start. But if I was ever going to be independent again, then this was the first step on that journey.

I took a cloth soaked in warm water and laid it over my legs. The water trickled over my shin and down onto the towel beneath me. I felt nothing. Little goosebumps prickled up on my thighs, rising up to tell me the water was felt, but, just as I had read, my brain couldn't register whether the cloth was warm or cold or my pressure too soft or too hard. My skin glistened. I crossed to the other leg, leaning forward for the first time, testing the limits of my reach. Stars filled my vision so I sat back and rested for a breath or two, leaving the water on my legs to dry in the air. I placed the cloth on my belly, it flinched but I felt nothing. The water trickled down into my groin. I saw that my pubic hair had regrown. Yellow stains of iodine discoloured my groin. I looked like a cadaver. But no matter how far I was tempted to go, nothing could bring me to touch in-between my legs. A urine tube came out from beneath me, but again, I held back. I didn't want to know what I could or could not feel there. Instead, I travelled upwards. Suddenly, I felt the cloth. Chilled by the air, the cold material rubbed the skin on my breasts. Topping up the warm water with another dunk, I returned the cloth to my chest and let the heat soak into me. As I moved the warm wet cloth up to my neck and down over my arms, trickles of water escaped down the crevices of my body, getting lost just as they fell into the grooves of my ribcage. I dunked it again and then squeezed the water out on to my chest, watching as it disappeared. Then I did it again with my eyes closed and felt where it disappeared.

An invisible line wrapped around me, an inch below the soft underneath of my breasts.

I tried to trace it.

I could feel the warmth of myself, the tiny fluffy baby hairs and the goosebumps, but if I closed my eyes the feedback came only from my hand, not from what my hand touched. Touching myself below the level was like touching someone else.

I prodded my belly, pinched my thighs, scratched my shins as though they weren't mine.

I had read in the manual that some people with spinal cord injury often think of themselves as having two birthdays: their actual birthday and the day they were injured. Some call this a 'Life Day'. It's not unusual, therefore, when asked how old you are, to give two ages.

I was eighteen.

And I was one month old.

Disabled Rage

Until this point, visitors had been restricted to a handful of carefully selected close family friends, but as my face began to heal, I began to sit up, my need for morphine lessened, and my energy levels started to even out, my thoughts turned once again to my friends. I missed them all.

'Mum,' I asked one morning as she arrived looking flustered and tired as always. 'Would it be possible to get in touch with Boner, Sophia and Ellie? I'd really love to see them. And do you think maybe you could call Jack?'

'Phie?' she said, tilting her head in a sort of pitiful but sympathetic nod. 'Don't you remember seeing any of them? Well, apart from Jack. The girls have all been here to see you; I just haven't really let them visit too often because I know that you've had so much to deal with. I thought maybe it was best to wait until you were ready. But they've been here all along. That loony Antonia, or Boner as you call her, has been coming down from Scotland every week; sweet little Sophia has been here too. And gorgeous Ellie. Not every day, but near enough. And then some of your friends from King's, and of course darling Anna and Phoebe and some of your other friends from home. They all sit outside on the grassy bank together, everybody smoking and hugging each other.'

If my mouth could have fallen open, it would have.

'After your injury,' she continued, 'the police handed back your phone to us. Tom called through your entire contact list and told every single one of your friends what had happened. Most of them seemed to have dropped what they were doing and come straight here. I have to say, one of the only silver linings about this whole fucking nightmare is getting to spend time with all of your friends.'

I don't know what shocked me more – the fact my little brother had been so strong, or that my friends were all outside, or the fact that I didn't remember seeing any of them.

'The girls are dying to see you again,' Mum said. 'We've been waiting for you to ask and we didn't want to overwhelm you. Also, Jack hasn't been able to come down' – I saw a flicker of rage in her eyes – 'but he sent your mutual friend Alick to help us out. When he turned up at home, he gave me and your dad the fright of our lives, fucking enormous bloke, isn't he! With that skinhead.' She laughed fondly. 'He looks like he eats babies for breakfast. But honestly, he has been such a godsend. Helping out at home when I am here and your dad's at work, walking the dogs while Tom's at school, stocking the fridge . . .'

Mum had been right, this was too overwhelming.

A heart-stopping thought flashed through my mind momentarily. Had Rory been called, and if so what had his response been?

'There's something else I've been meaning to tell you.' I braced myself. I was bracing myself a lot; I'd never done so much bloody bracing of myself. But Mum was elated; in fact, she appeared so happy she reminded me of the last time I had seen her smiling so honestly, when I hadn't waved goodbye.

'So, we didn't tell you, but the day you went up to the party, we got a new dog. We'd just got him home the night the call came, so we had to give him back to his breeder. But we got him back last week and, well, would you like to meet him soon? You just can't tell Gary or anyone, as we aren't technically allowed to have puppies in the hospital, but your dad and I have got a plan.'

It was all too much. My mum, plotting with my dad. A new puppy. My friends. My family.

I don't think I've ever felt so much gratitude in my life.

A few days later Gary popped his head around the door.

'Look what I've just found . . . '

Boner leapt out from behind him.

'Ta da!' She threw out her hands dramatically, but then caught herself. 'Oh my fuck—'

'It's all right, Antonia . . . ' Gary did his best to cover up her shock, gathering her up and walking her towards me. He pulled up a chair beside my bed and plonked her on it. 'She's been trying to get to see you but your mum said it would be best to wait a bit. She's introduced herself to all of us nurses, though, haven't you, lovey?'

'Oh, Morgan . . . ' Boner said quietly, our first words in this new reality. 'What have you *done* to yourself?'

For the very first time since I'd regained consciousness, I wanted to laugh out loud. I couldn't take my eyes off her. She looked tanned and healthy. Her hair had been cut short, and it gave her a dramatic look, especially with her multicoloured dungarees. She belonged in the spotlight, on the stage, not here, with me.

Gary put an arm on her shoulder. 'Sophie's doing incredibly well, aren't you, princess? She's washing herself.'

'Well, that's a first,' laughed Boner hard, one of my most favourite sounds, 'she hardly bothered to wash herself even when she could bloody walk!' Never one for sitting down for long, Boner jumped up and started checking out my room. She felt so close yet there was this vast distance between us. The smell of her was so familiar it made me woozy. I tried to reach out for her hand.

'Morg! Look at all your cards and flowers. You are *loved,* you know. Look – a postcard from Celia! *"We've arrived in Australia safe and sound. Having the best time, but thinking of you always."* Lucky thing. Such a relief she only had that head wound, isn't it? Oh, don't you wish you could be in Australia right now? Hey, look, a note from Jack's parents.'

I couldn't listen to her talking about the passengers in the car. I didn't have the capacity to think about them as well as my family. I couldn't face up to how many people I had hurt.

I deliberately hadn't asked for my phone back, or for anyone to read me the cards that sat in piles on the sides and were displayed on the walls, so I could try to hide from how much of a mess I'd made.

'Have you heard from Jack?' she asked without realising what she was doing to me. 'Or Rory?'

It was only a few days ago that I had started to piece together where everyone was. The news that she and so many others had been there all along had rattled me, but to know my friendships had been tested and passed felt like a badge of honour. For a moment, I had felt proud, but then the uneasiness that followed consumed me. *Why hadn't Jack come down?* And there was no mention of Rory.

The two boys felt more important to me than ever before, and yet just like Boner was, they felt out of my reach. But the more I thought about their absence the more hurt I felt.

I sucked some water through my clenched jaws. It was all I could do to stop the additional excruciating pain in my chest that contained my deeper fear that, like *this*, I would be rejected by them anyway.

It felt safer to just put thoughts of them both in a box in my mind and lock them away for now, and I decided I certainly didn't want my phone back any time soon. At least with it off, I wouldn't know who *wasn't* trying to contact me.

Thankfully at that moment, Mum arrived.

'Bone!' Mum rushed over to give my friend a hug. 'I didn't know you were down again, darling girl. That's so good of you.' She released her from her hug. 'Morning, Phie.' She looked at me. 'How are you today?'

'Gary says she's making amazing progress, Carol.' Boner came over to me, and to my delight I got to hold her hand. She squeezed it back with all she had.

'You are so thin, Soph,' she said, her thumb and index finger wrapped around my wrist to make a bracelet, which she ran up my forearm. 'I've never seen you so thin. And look at your beautiful face . . . ' She stroked my hair and tidied up the strays around my wounds. 'Oh Soph . . . '

'Honestly, this is nothing, Antonia. You should have seen her when she was first admitted in Scotland. Her face was in pieces. But they've done such a great job patching her up, haven't they? I mean, your nose will have to be reconstructed a few more times, Phie, but we'll cross that bridge when we have to. It was touch and go for a while, as you know, Bone, but she's still here, aren't you, Phie Phie Trixibelle—'

Mum's voice broke ever so slightly, and Bone rushed over to her, enveloping her in a hug.

'Carol, we are here for you too, you know? You mustn't feel that you are on your own.' Mum's posture softened in Bone's hug. 'Shall we go for a cig, Carol? Come on, let's go outside for a smoke.'

Watching my friend walk the despondent frame of my mother outside, a deeply unsettling, unfamiliar and unbearable feeling crept up on me, like a cold sweat.

Was this jealousy? I was deeply grateful to Bone for the kindness she was showing my mum, but it was muddled in with resentment of her being able to be with Mum when I wanted more than anything to be the one to hug her and shield her from this terror; to distract her from the reality I had created for her. That was *my* job. But instead, I was the monster from whom she needed rescuing and I couldn't stand up to rescue her.

I felt the wrath of pure *disabled rage* for the first time, and it was so disturbing I reached out and held on to the side of the bed. *Steady, steady*, I whispered to myself, but the rage was so strong, I couldn't control myself. I broke down, tearing out my stitches as my face contracted in heartache. The tears loosened my scabs and every thought from the parts of my mind I had shut out came gushing forward.

I wept fully and desperately, for everything I had heard, seen and read so far. I wept in fear for all of the unknown that was yet to come, I wept for my friends and for my family, who I pictured clinging to one another outside in a fog of smoke.

And I wept because I had no idea how to find the strength to keep going.

What Matters Most

I could paint you a portrait from memory of the people who looked after me during that time, they are that vivid to me still. Gary, with his rounded face, always had rosy cheeks. He had thin lips, a wide smile, black ink tattooed on his arms, and a white nurse's uniform. Emma, with brown-blonde cropped hair, a tall thin masculine frame, and a friendly but uncompromising look on her face. Debbie, short and sweet, with her round brown eyes and tidy blonde hair, in a blue uniform.

But the face of the inpatient mental health counsellor would be just an abstract blur, a flick of brown for hair and a splash of red for lipstick maybe, because she never sat long enough for me to know what she looked like. When she visited my hospital bed I didn't know how to speak about what had happened to me, especially to a person who themselves had never experienced being paralysed. The idea of risking confessing my deepest darkest fears out loud, to a stranger, only to get back platitudes felt potentially more traumatising than trying to replay the car crash itself. I guessed Mum must have told her, in her typically blunt and unmindful way, that 'we don't do depression' or words to that effect because I never saw her again, nor did I ask for her.

Instead, I asked Mum to get me a diary to document what was happening to me, and already one step ahead, she pulled out a black leather journal that she had bought not long after I had been admitted to the spinal unit. This had shaken me a little at first, all of my diaries from my girlhood were colourful, but the one Mum had selected was plain and nondescript. To me, it was the journal of a grown-up and whether or not it was chosen deliberately to encourage me to be one, somehow it did.

My diary became the outlet for my thoughts, and I unloaded everything on to its pages. To release some of the more painful or haunting images from my mind I would close my eyes and put my pen on the page, and then draw blindly from my imagination. I'd open my eyes to see the figures had come out dancing, jumping and hugging, but also screaming, trying to fly and wrapped up in themselves; small single figures alone on the floor, their heads pressed into their hands.

I hid the diary under my pillow so that no one would find it and see what a state I was really in.

There was another person whose face I don't recall clearly, but who I remember because of how awful she made me feel. This was a nurse who one morning came into my room and closed the door behind her, twisting the blinds closed with a slap. Unlike so many of the nurses who came in and out of my room, I didn't recognise her, and she, and her box marked 'sharps and disposables', put me on edge instantly. Without introduction, she marched around the room, tutting at the clutter and looking for somewhere to perch. She decided my bed would be suitable and with one white-gloved scoop, dragged my legs to one side to make room for herself.

'Morning. I'm here to teach you how to catheterise.'

Everything in me flipped upside down. I had no idea how to respond.

'Okay, I will explain this to you and then will assist you whilst you have a go yourself. Don't worry if you don't get the hang of this at first, it can be complicated for people with vulvas.'

Tight-lipped, the woman spread a square plastic-lined mat on to the bed, neatly arranging a selection of objects into sharp lines. She then talked me through her medical picnic spread.

'This long clear tube is a catheter,' she said, pointing to it as if it were an option on one of those restaurant dessert trollies. 'It's sterilised so that you don't get an infection when you insert it, and comes in a sleeve that once opened must be thrown away along with the used catheter.'

My stomach lurched as I recognised it from the manual.

'Here we have soap and water to wash your hands, and this container is for you to empty into. I see you have a mirror already, that'll be very useful.' She handed me the mirror and motioned for where I should look. 'You may have noticed you have an indwelling catheter that is draining into a urine bag. That's fine for now, but seeing as you have full function in your hands, we advise that you learn how to *self*-catheterise, which is shorthand for inserting a catheter into your bladder every few hours to manually drain yourself. Some paraplegics ...' she continued, with a momentary hesitation that made me look up at her, 'choose to keep a urine bag in, all the time, but we suggest you learn to self-catheterise. We've already started you on medication that will help your bladder to retain fluid, and prevent leaks between self-catheterising, but as everyone's bladder is different, you'll have to learn how much you can drink and what types of beverages might cause you to have an accident.' I looked away. 'But, seeing as you will be doing this every day for the rest of your life, we're sure you'll get to know just how to look after yourself best. The issue with having a complete spinal cord injury of your level is that you'll not know *when* you need to empty your bladder, or bowels, so you have to gauge this yourself. Sounds daunting now but over time you'll hopefully begin noticing your body sending you alternative signals that warn you. Some people get headaches, others sweat, it all depends. We call this autonomic dysreflexia.' I recognised this term from the manual. 'When you get a urine infection or your bowels are blocked, for example, same with if you injure yourself, then your body may send you signals. You are at the beginning of your journey, so we won't know what these signals are *just* yet.'

Finally, she stopped speaking. I'd experienced some of the less amenable nurses, but this one really was unaware of the impact of the words she was saying. Or, maybe she was doing her job and the disconnect was on my side, petrified about what I was about to learn.

'So,' she was ready to continue, 'you'll have to open your legs and position your hips so that you can feel for the entry to the urethra in your vulva, and then once you've identified the correct hole you insert the catheter up your urinary tract and into the bladder which will then empty either into this container or, when you are eventually able to transfer, into the toilet.'

I let the nurse begin the process of moving my legs into position as I wasn't strong enough to lift them by myself. Silently, I washed and dried my hands and then she handed me the mirror.

'Have you ever looked at yourself down there before?'

I nodded.

'Great, well, this won't be so hard for you. Some women have literally never looked at themselves so this can be a little intense. You aren't wearing underwear, are you? No, great, okay. So get in a position where you are able to see yourself in the mirror. Do you need a hand?' She put another pillow under my leg. 'Right,' she said, 'next get your mirror and look at your vulva, then you need to part your labia and, using your mirror, have a look to see where the tube of your current indwelling catheter enters. Can you see?' I nodded. 'Okay, so we are going to take that out now and I'll come back in a few hours, enough time to fill your bladder up.' I watched the mirror as she pulled out the tube from my bladder. 'Good,' she said, and handed me a glass of water. 'Drink this and the rest of that jug, and I'll be back soon to teach you the rest.'

When she left, I sat silently for a moment, my eyes closed and my head rolled back.

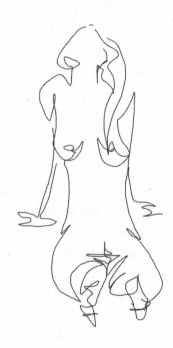

After a moment, I brought my mind back to focus on what was happening, pinching my thigh to remind myself that was happening to me, was without doubt, real. My leg didn't respond, but, regardless, I knew there was no hiding from what I had just learned, my deepest fear had just been realised; just like my legs and my stomach, I was unable to feel every part of my lower body.

I closed my eyes and hugged myself.

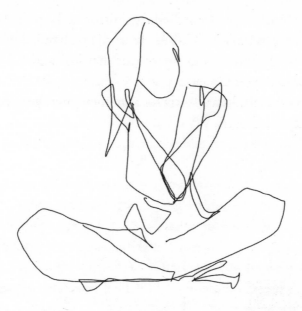

An hour later the nurse returned. I felt as though I was hanging over the edge of a cliff, dangling by my fingertips and she was about to stamp on them. She got straight back to work.

'Okay, let's get your mirror again and this time I'll show you how to put this,' she picked up another instrument from the dessert trolley of torture, '"intermittent catheter" in. These are the ones you use once and throw away, the ones you'll be using from now on. Right. You ready, Sophie? I'll hold the mirror this time and you can do it for yourself.' She handed it to me. My hands were shaking. I had never been so quiet in my life, but what was there to say?

'Feel for the hole just above the entrance to your vagina.' She watched as my fingers stumbled. 'That's it, a little higher, there – now hold one hand there and insert the catheter. Excellent. Now, here we are, use the container . . .'

I looked between my thighs and a trickle of urine ran out of the tube and turned the cardboard dark as it filled up.

'Well done!'

The container filled and a faint whiff of ammonia filled the air.

'Now that's finished, give a little cough to ensure it's all out,' she said, unbothered by the smell. 'Oh sorry, as best as you can with your jaw like that. Well done, now squeeze the end, pull it out, and there we go. Wasn't too painful, was it?'

My hands were trembling so much I nearly dropped the container.

I shook no, and closed my eyes again, thinking that it wasn't *painful* because I couldn't *feel* it. I still couldn't speak.

'Right,' she said obliviously. 'Good work, Sophie. Now, remind me. Have you reached the part in your rehabilitation education about sexual function yet?'

'No. Not yet.' I didn't move; my face must have turned white despite all the bruises.

'Right, well,' she said as she busied herself, tidying up all the pissing paraphernalia, 'that's pretty straightforward too. Technically you can still have it, but you won't *feel* it. There should be something about this in your SCI manual. Okay, well done.' She smiled and left.

At these words, as though she had punched me in the stomach, I lost my breath.

Breathless and still trembling, I touched myself again.

I couldn't feel my touch.

I couldn't feel *myself.*

But, if I can't *feel* myself, how can I ever feel *myself* ever again?

I touched my pubic hair and stroked the hair on my legs. I noticed someone had trimmed my toenails, but, I thought, *how can things grow where there's no life?*

I had known all along that this was coming, but denial and ignorance had felt like safer ground to hold. When I was in denial I didn't feel as though I might stop breathing altogether.

I looked down at my paralysed body.

Will I never again have the key to access my own body? At that moment, I didn't care about not knowing when I needed to urinate, not knowing if I could feel hot or cold, pain or pressure. *What if I could no longer feel* pleasure?

I tried to recall the sensation of arousal between my legs. I pictured myself lying in my school uniform, my tights ripped open, spread out on the ground underneath a green canopy of trees overhead, Jack kissing me, the two of us lost deep in the woods in our favourite spot. His hand in me, his tongue on me, him inside me.

I felt my face flush red, but below me, silence.

I tried again.

I squeezed my eyes and thought back for the hottest memory I could find. There I was, with Jack, behind a locked door, in one of the boarding houses at school. His face was between my legs; I was standing over him.

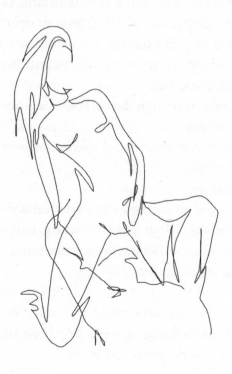

As I thought of him bringing me to orgasm, my breath quickened, but still, nothing below my breasts responded.

This. Cannot. Be. Happening.

From the moment I'd started having sex with Jack, when I was fifteen years old, I knew that there was nothing in the world to beat it. I knew I'd discovered the one act that could calm me down, that could reach the unsatisfied rage in me. In sex, all of the longing and animal hunger I'd always had was finally fed. But I was never able to get full; I wanted feeding again every fucking day.

So what now? Would it only be me inside myself now, just me, and an empty space? Before I could stop myself, I thought back to the night of the crash. I thought about Rory standing by the car. I thought about how ferociously I'd driven. I thought about my drive for sex. Then I thought about my reckless behaviour throughout my life. I thought back to every time I'd been naughty, ruthless and selfish. I thought about my urgency to race into my life. The destruction I'd left in my wake now seemed to be drowning me. A tsunami of guilt slammed down on me and shame settled like toxic sediment over my lifeless limbs. I reached under my pillow and took out my diary thinking the universe must be trying to tell me that whatever force had been driving me was wrong. That enough was enough. I was too much. *Why else would this have happened to me?* I mean, surely there could have been other, less drastic ways for me to have learnt my lesson? *Taking away the sensation from my body,* I scribbled frantically. *The universe isn't that much of a cunt, is she?*

Of all the things that I'd lost, I knew then that not being able to walk would matter to me the least.

Not here

After I had learnt the full extent of my paralysis, something in me broke. Something as damaging as my broken spine. Reality had hit me hard, and any hopes I had harboured for a return to normal had now vanished. I had been in hospital just over a month and had made progress through the manual, but learning to catheterise felt like one step forward and an infinite number back.

But rehabilitation didn't stop. As the wounds on my face mended, it seemed everyone assumed I was mentally healing too. But internally, I was fractured, part of me pushing forward, the other part giving up.

Mum was still living in the nurses' quarters so that she could be close to me. Her omnipresence was reassuring, but the guilt I experienced at the sight of her overwhelmed me. I had hurt Mum plenty of times over the years, and let her down countless more, but I'd never felt any real lasting remorse. She had always been strong enough to brush off whatever I threw at her. The drinking, the rebellion, the suspensions and then expulsions from school hadn't hurt her, they'd angered her. I'd felt frightened of her rage before, but what was happening between us in the hospital was entirely different. She looked destroyed. It was hard to stomach.

I was almost relieved that Dad's work was keeping him busy, because I didn't feel I had the strength to look at him either, or my brother, who thankfully had gone back to boarding school. My friends came in to see me, bringing me mix tapes, leaving me with equally mixed emotions. Of them all, Alick and the three girls made the most time for me, but soon they would be starting work or going to university. Their lives were taking off.

I now understood that my spine had been irreparably damaged, with no chance of recovery, and the consequence – complete paralysis – was far more complicated than I could have ever imagined, and although my education was being expertly guided by the manual and my team, most of the facts were failing to sink in.

Every day my consultant stopped by my room, to check my progress and check with Gary that I was where I should be in the rehabilitation journey. I would give him a fake smile and long to be anywhere else. But how long I would be in the hospital was one question I could not get an answer to. I had to complete my education before they would even entertain a conversation about when I might be able to go home. Going home was all I wanted, and yet, what I was going home to was equally unclear. It struck me that this motivation was so different to what had been driving me forward only a matter of weeks ago; I had been ready to leave home and never look back, but now, it was the only place I wanted to be.

The most important part of rehabilitation was looming and my team excitedly assured me that this next step would be pivotal, would feel like progress, but who on earth looks forward to the day when they are going to get into a wheelchair for the first time?

*

'Today's the day, Soph.' Gary positioned himself at the end of my bed some days later. 'It's time to get you sitting in a wheelchair, darling.'

Mum, who had been sitting quietly beside me reading my medical notes, put them down and looked at Gary over her glasses. 'Don't worry, Carol, babe, we've consulted with the Consultant Gods above, and it has been agreed that Sophie is ready. So, give me a moment, and we'll get going. I just have to go find Emma, okay, princess?' Gary gave me his best spin and exited through the curtain dramatically.

I laughed, but this might have been the most unfunny thing anyone had ever said to me in my life. Ever. Reading my mind, Mum rolled her eyes in sympathy and returned to reading my notes. I looked out of the window and hoped I wouldn't pass out.

Emma came in pushing a rigid-framed aluminium wheelchair with a black cushion. Gary was beaming at me. This was a milestone of a moment according to the manual and my team, but I was still reeling from the catheter experience. I assessed the wheelchair, which was frayed and battered and looked as though a good many people had sat in it before me. I wondered if they had been shitting themselves as much as I was. I looked for stains. *Seems clean enough.*

With nothing in the manual about how to *mentally* approach sitting in a wheelchair for the first time, I had picked Gary's brains in the days before. He told me there was a chance my blood pressure could drop, but I had been sitting up and washing myself. I was ready, he insisted. And yet, I wasn't so sure.

Once again, my thoughts strayed to the other 'me'. *My life isn't supposed to be like this.*

Emma began to gently position a hoist underneath me. She rolled me to one side, tucked the brown fabric underneath me and then carefully rolled me back towards her so she could straighten out the bunched-up material below me. Once she had arranged me on top of the hoist material, she rolled the stand over to the bed and fixed the brakes.

No one spoke, including me. I watched Emma clicking the material into the straps of the hoist. I could smell cigarettes on her breath. She winked at me. The wounds in my face began to pulsate with my heartbeat. I looked around the room. Gary, Mum and Debbie stood near me, watching. I wondered if they all felt heightened awareness of their legs at that moment? *Are you consciously flexing your calf muscles right now?* I thought. *Are you squeezing your thigh muscles? Tensing your butt? Wriggling your toes? Reminding yourselves what your bodies can do?*

I looked at my feet: Mum had slipped them into some trainers for the occasion. The trainers were brand new. *They'll never get dirty with me as their owner,* I thought to myself.

Doing so little to move myself, myself, was bizarre.

Being so passive I felt as damaged as I had ever known.

I wondered how Mum could stomach watching this happen, witnessing me returning to such an infantile state, but she seemed as strong as ever, and even stepped forward to ask Emma if she needed a hand with the hoist.

'Right then,' Emma said after she had checked everything was in place.

I avoided eye contact with them all, and just looked into the middle distance between us all. *Breathe.*

'Okay, Em,' I said. 'Let's do this.'

Emma clicked a button and the hoist started to engage.

Suddenly, Mum let out a horrible yelp.

'Jack!'

'Hello?' A thin, scared Scottish voice came through the doorway of the ward. 'Hello? Is Sophie Morgan in here?'

'Jack!' Mum rushed towards Jack's voice, looking to me for guidance on what the fuck to do with him. The horror-struck look on my face must have told her I wasn't ready to see him. That, or I was about to faint.

'Hi, Carol.' Jack was now coming towards the bay, but before he could enter Mum ushered him away, and, swooping up behind her, Gary quickly closed the door.

'Sorry, love, let's keep visitors out for now.'

Everyone looked at me. I was shaken to my broken core. I could hear Mum outside the bay telling Jack to go and get a drink and wait. I could hear his deep voice murmuring in reply. I wondered if she was thinking what I once thought about Ellie and her disabled boyfriend: he'd better not *hurt* her.

The door reopened and Mum came back in. I felt as though I had left my body and was watching this play out from above. My legs were scrunched up in the hoist and all eyes were on me. I hung suspended over my bed.

'Phie, are you okay?' Mum asked, rushing over to me.

'Are you okay, Soph?'

'Princess, are you okay?'

NO! I screamed inside. *No. No. No. Not now, not here, not like this! He can't see me like this, the broken Sophie, he isn't looking for her.*

The team was poised, watching and waiting for my instruction.

Fuck it.

I nodded back.

'I'm okay, yes I am OKAY.' I blocked him out of my mind. 'Keep going please ...'

Emma checked the position of the hoist and everyone held their breath once more. The whirring sound of the hoist kicked in and I watched as my body was gathered up and lifted out of the bed completely. Once I was high enough for clearance, they pivoted me around, swung me directly over the wheelchair and started to lower me down.

Thump. I landed.

Looking down I could see that I was now sitting within the frame of the giant wheelchair, but without any sensation to tell me where my body was it felt like I was floating on air. My brain whirred in confusion, like a car engine in the wrong gear.

The team began to release the clips from the hoist so I would be free to move. The new trainers dangled below me. I leant forward to position my feet on the footplate of the chair, but unable to engage my core muscles, I lost my balance.

'Emma!'

'Christ, careful, Soph.' Emma grabbed my shoulders and yanked me upright. Stars filled my eyes.

'This is the strangest ...' I didn't know what to say. With no core to hold me upright, my stomach felt deflated, and the breath fell out of me. My face pounded.

'Water please,' I said dizzily. Gary was already walking towards me with a glass and straw.

'Go slowly, darling. You will get very lightheaded when you first sit up, remember? Just breathe and *go slow*.' What the fuck did he think I was about to do? *Go running?* I had never moved so slowly in my life! I sucked up some water and looked at Mum.

'Can I take Sophie outside?' Mum's question to Emma scared the crap out of me. Mum didn't need permission to move me. Did *I* need someone to move me?

'Great idea, Carol!' Gary rushed to move all the furniture out of my path so I could cross the room and go out through the door into the garden.

Mum went behind me and, as if pushing her baby in a pram again, took me out to see the world.

I'd been dreaming of being outside in the fresh air for weeks, but now that I was outside, I wanted nothing more than to go back in.

'Are you okay, Phie?' she asked me softly.

The wheelchair wobbled underneath me, and I felt turbulence rattle through the parts of my body that I could feel. Movement reverberated up through the metalwork in my face. That was the only sensation I could decipher in the movement, my face connecting me to the ground. I looked down and nowhere else.

The sunshine outside felt as blinding and unwelcoming as bright lights in an operating theatre. I winced and felt the stitches on my face pull and throb. Fresh, soft air tickled the hair on my arms and goosebumps appeared, but not on the pinch of belly that poked out below my arms. I touched my skin there but still felt nothing. With my stomach muscles no longer engaged, the flat stroke of my belly was gone. Looking down at it, it looked punctured, the air let out of the firm rigid tyre it once had been. Soft and useless, my core couldn't hold me up. The ground wobbled and so did my thighs. These sections of my body had once been solid to touch, the muscles defined by years of running and swimming, but they had wasted away so rapidly, and instead I sat on a soft seat of podge that jiggled as I moved over the ground.

I couldn't take my eyes off the pavement, every single crack was enough to interrupt the flow of the wheels on the chair and, so confused was my brain by this whole sensation, I felt lifted out of my body again.

'Phie?' Mum asked.

I nodded and kept my hands folded in my lap.

And then, out of the corner of my eye, I saw him. Jack. He was watching me through a window, smiling the smile that had, for so many years, been reserved for me. The face I would catch watching me in lessons or spying on me through the window of the art block. Whenever I would catch his eyes on me, I would break out smiling in return and run towards him, but at the sight of him now I instantly felt the exact opposite. I wanted to run away. He smiled at me and lifted a hand in hello. A wave that implied *don't worry about anything any more, I am here.*

Suddenly, though, I saw what he was looking at. Thick white hospital stockings on my atrophied legs. Unfitted stained grey tracksuit crumpled up around my waist. A thin filthy nude-pink T-shirt hung over my braless chest. The protruding paunch of my stomach poking from below my top. The wide clunky metal frame of the hospital wheelchair caging me. My rings were gone. My bracelets, too. And my face. I couldn't even think about my face. My jaw pounded and one eye seeped with fluid. I reached up to touch my thickly matted hair. I felt grit in my scalp still.

Mum let go of the handles of the chair and walked around to crouch down to hear me, and as soon as she let go the chair lurched forward, stopping abruptly on a small crack in the pavement. 'Mum ... *Please* ... ' I couldn't be there any more. I started to well up.

'Oh Phie, not here. Not here. Let me take you back inside. Gary!' Mum cried. 'Gary, please help me get Sophie back inside.'

The moment I was back in bed and the hoist and wheelchair had been removed from my room, Mum closed everyone out.

The image of myself in the wheelchair ...

I am the girl in the manual, I realised.

She is me.

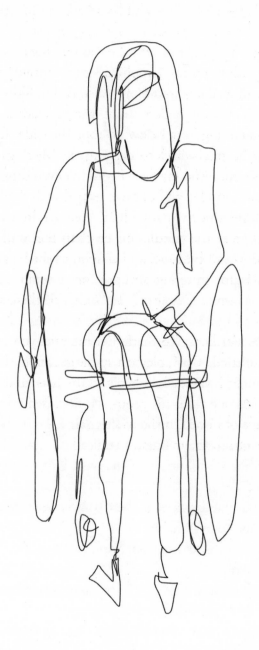

Held

Later that day, Jack sat on the end of my hospital bed, my paralysed feet on his lap. As much as I had wanted to see him, his unexpected arrival had completely unravelled me. He smiled at me as he stroked my feet, and I didn't know how to tell him I wanted him to stop. We had been alone for two minutes. I looked again at the clock. Three minutes. Every wound on my face throbbed as I flushed, embarrassed by what I must look like to him, *like a fucking car crash*. I put thoughts of my appearance to one side.

'It's good to see you, Jack . . .' This was only partly true. Him looking at me so closely was uncomfortable, and looking back at him felt like wandering into the past, which would not end well for me.

I looked at the clock and then back at my feet. I tried to wiggle my toes, out of habit.

'Aye, it's good to see you too, Soph.'

'How are you?'

'You don't need to talk, if it hurts your jaws? Your face looks so painful. Is it painful? Are you in pain?'

I shrugged, and showed him the morphine clicker. 'Morphine helps.'

Jack fingered the clicker and his flexing calloused hands

made my memory banks begin to open. I quickly slammed them shut.

'What happened, Jack? Where have you been since ... since ...?' I trailed off, uncertain of what I wanted to call that night. The accident, the car crash, the night I nearly died.

'What do you remember, Soph?' I shrugged to say not much, and braced myself for whatever he was about to tell me. I was curious about the details but worried about the impact they might have.

'Well, after the party, we all drove back to Rory's house.'

At the mention of Rory's name coming from Jack's mouth, my stomach flipped. Jack would not have known about my intentions for that night, and even though, in the end, nothing had happened, hearing him mention Rory somehow still felt like a betrayal. Jack had been my partner for so long, and any issues that once existed between us seemed almost childish in the presence of a life-changing injury. We were kids before. We were something else now. With him finally in front of me, selfishly I also realised just how much I needed his help.

'After we left the party,' Jack continued, 'I was sitting behind you, Rory in the passenger seat, his brother and Celia in the back with me. You were driving so fast, and the music was so loud. We raced down the road parallel to the runway, and then you misjudged a corner and I couldn't see what happened exactly but suddenly the car flipped into the field, we rolled for ages. When the car stopped, we were upside down. Rory climbed out of the passenger window and the rest of us climbed out of the back window. You were trapped. Rory stayed talking to you, while I called for an ambulance. Celia was screaming, she had a cut on her head ...' Everything he was describing felt imagined. I couldn't recall most of it. 'After you were taken to hospital,' Jack continued, 'another ambulance came to get the rest of us. The police were sniffing around, trying to accuse you of drink-driving, but you were breathalysed and they went away, I think. It was a bit of a blur after the shock, to be honest. Anyway, my parents came to get me and I went home. The next thing I heard was that you were flown south. I stayed at home in Scotland, as I had work. I really wanted to come down and see you. I just needed some time to deal with it all . . . ' He paused. 'Do *you* remember what happened that night?'

I shook my head, watching him still stroking my feet, wishing it was soothing but it was having the opposite effect.

'Well, I do,' he continued, his facial expression almost unrecognisable, 'I remember everything and I haven't been able to sleep since. But look, let's not talk about all that for now. I just want to be here for you, in whatever way I can. I know that we were planning to break up – we basically did that night, if you remember – but I love you, Soph, very much.'

Looking up from my feet, I met his eyes properly.

'I love you too.' At that moment, I wanted to be anywhere else but in that room. I wanted to be with him, just the two of us, in the woods in Scotland, in our own world. I was so grateful to see him I could barely speak.

'I'm staying with my sister in London for the moment, so I can visit you anytime you like,' he said.

The stitches on my face started to itch. I reached up to tentatively scratch one and Jack leant in and stroked my cheek softly. With his hands where I could feel them, he instantly felt real.

'Can I hug you?' he asked. 'Would that be okay? I don't want to hurt you.'

'Yes, *please* . . . '

He stood and re-placed my feet carefully on the bed, then he came around the side of me, and scooped me up under my knees and around my back. Like a hoist, he picked me up a few centimetres from the mattress as slowly as he could, looking to me for reassurance. I nodded to tell him I was fine. Aside from my face aching, the movement didn't hurt my back or any other part of my body I was able to feel. Being so close to him, and in his arms in this way, completely calmed me down, but I felt more self-conscious than I imagined possible.

Having shuffled me a few centimetres over, he climbed on to the bed beside me. He tucked one arm behind my neck, and wrapped the other around me. He had never been so careful with me before. He treated me as I had treated myself, like a newborn baby. He kissed the sections of my face that weren't damaged. He even kissed my lips, although my mouth remained wired closed and I longed to kiss him back.

But with him so close to me, I soon became unglued. The chasm between our realities opened wider with every kiss. I didn't know how much he knew about my spinal injury, whether or not anyone had told him what my paralysis had done to my body. He would have known that I was unable to walk, but I was unsure how much more he knew. Had any of my family or friends explained anything about catheters or bowel management? Did he know that I couldn't feel his arm as it rested across my stomach? Didn't he know I wasn't able to feel my feet when he stroked them, not *at all*? *Was he hoping I might?*

Jack touched the cannula in my hand, then stopped moving, and settled down. The familiar smell of his aftershave reached my new nose and I wanted to retch and smile at the same time.

'Thank you for being here with me,' I whispered.

'You don't need to thank me.' His blue eyes met mine.

'But I mean it, I am thankful. I love you so much. I am so sorry . . .'

'You don't need to apologise. What has happened has happened. You just need to focus on getting stronger, Soph.'

'Jack, when you look at me do you still see me? Do you see *me*?' My voice broke. In the unspoken conversation that we were having, I begged him to say, *Yes*.

'What do you mean? *Of course* I do. You will always be *you*.'

But as soon as he said it I got angry. His answer, like my question, sounded naive and unconsidered.

'How do you *know* that?' All of the talking was taking its toll on my jaw. I pressed on the morphine clicker. Jack could see I was irritated but couldn't understand what he had done wrong.

'I just mean that ... you will always ... be *you*.' He squeezed me in his arms and kissed my forehead. But Jack had no idea what he was saying and the confidence with which he was speaking insulted me. I noticed, however, that feeling defensive of myself, feeling angry, fighting back, felt surprisingly refreshing. I had been consumed with dread, guilt, sadness and fear for so long, anger, my old default emotion, felt great, and whether he meant to or not, Jack had just given me back a little part of myself.

Letting the matter go, I leant towards him and put my lips on his. I asked him to change the subject and tell me about something else. We stayed cuddled together and he told me about his family and how his work had been, and I listened, feeling strangely motivated. Rage simmered under the surface of me like a shield.

But that shield could only withstand so much.

Watching him walk away from me that evening, I suddenly remembered the happiness and excitement of running up behind him and jumping on his back as he played among a crowd of friends at school, a head taller than everyone; the sound of his laughter as he clasped my legs around his waist to spin me around and around; the way I'd jump down off him as I pulled one of his hands towards me, wrapping his arm over my shoulder like a scarf so I could walk beside him so close and warm. His mouth was the perfect height to kiss my forehead as we walked, my arm wrapped around his waist. This was how we had walked through our lives together, not one in front of the other or one below the other, but beside one another.

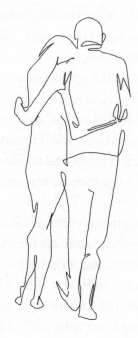

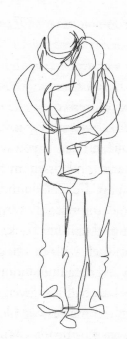

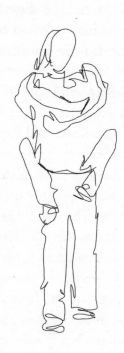

The rage and resolve had gone, and the anguish had taken its place. As he walked away, I dissolved into uncontrollable sobs, feeling more alone than I had ever known, alone to my core, alone in the deepest hollow in the shell of a body that couldn't even talk to itself.

Alone on my bed, I cried until I ran out of breath.

But as I clawed my way back, pulling myself together, I acknowledged that in order to avoid any more unbearable spirals into the past, I'd somehow have to learn how to protect myself from these unpredictable triggers.

I tried to think what else might trigger me: the first few beats of Aim's 'Cold Water Music', fresh air with tobacco smoke, Faithless, Underworld, Common, my name teased out slowly in a Scottish accent, the breeze through a birch tree forest. These little red buttons danced in my mind like the cherry cigarettes in the woods in Scotland, and I tried to gather them together safely to avoid having to bump into them again, and get burnt.

Eventually, I stopped crying, drew a notch in my diary to mark the second time I had broken down, dusted myself off, picked myself up and made a note to always look the other way whenever Jack left the room.

Take My Body Back

With Jack by my side, I felt revitalised and determined and I began to see my situation as a competition, in which adapting successfully was the ultimate aim and the prize would be independence, autonomy, freedom. I needed something to work towards and those things had always been my goals before my injury, and they still applied – just in a different way. And although building character had never been a drive of mine before, with no hope for any change in my paralysis I had no choice than to grow mentally instead.

My sessions with Emma intensified.

I felt as though I was in an infant's body, with the mind of a young adult, and approached each task as a problem to be solved or a goal to be reached. Still in the embryonic stage of rehabilitation, the steps were small at first. Learning to roll my body in bed, how to sit up without the support of the hospital bed, how to move my body correctly – so as not to disturb the new metalwork in my spine – lift my legs, stretch my ankles and then how to pull my tracksuit over them, bending down to reach my toes – bizarrely, they felt colder to touch than the rest of me – and I wondered if I would ever get used to sliding my feet into a pair of shoes and not knowing whether or not my toes were crunched up. I would collapse in half, and unfolding myself upright required every bit of strength I had. The lack of core strength made almost every move a test of balance and I tottered and flopped wildly around my bed.

In an ongoing attempt to reclaim my identity, I asked for some old clothes to be brought up, but when they arrived, they looked like the clothes of another woman. The paint stains on the jeans and little holes in the tops were like portals into another life. Each stain held a memory, and determined to stop myself from time travelling backwards, I gave many of them to my friends, and like donating to a charity shop, I wondered where they might be worn next. Seeing the girls in my flared baggy trousers and long summer dresses, I wondered how they had once hung so effortlessly on me. This floppy little body couldn't hold up the floaty summer rags that my toned figure once had. I wondered if a paralysed body would ever look so comfortable and relaxed in clothing. Would I ever feel comfortable and relaxed, for that matter? I knew I would need new clothes to wrap me up, keep me safe and perhaps suggest that underneath, everything was still functioning as usual. Nothing unusual to see here. At some point, I would have to repopulate my wardrobe, but what that wardrobe would include I had no idea. How should paralysed bodies dress? It made me stop and think when I saw other patients, like me, wearing trainers. *Why?* I thought. *Where are we running to? What are we* training *for?* My confusion was fuelled by my inability to envision what paralysed bodies could *do*. There was nothing in the manual about that. I was secure in the land of the grey tracksuit for now, but I had started imagining myself in the world, and the frumpy, grey, passive mess I was currently in didn't belong outside.

I asked Mum to help me untangle my hair, and having been bound tightly above my head, untouched for weeks, the effort took her over four hours. Sitting in front of her as she teased out my mane, the way she had once deloused me as a kid, I reflected on the fact that with no *body* to show off any more, my hair might come to matter to me more. Perhaps I would learn what to do with it, other than just tie it back and forget about it? Like writing in my plain black leather diary, thinking about hairstyles made me feel grown up.

As I progressed, Emma gave the green light for me to be hoisted into a wheelchair once a day, increasing the time I could sit up by an hour at a time, and as the days passed, I began to look forward to it. Getting out of my bed meant I could get my bearings in the ward, I could see the other patients and, most significantly, it meant I was one step closer to getting out of hospital.

The initial fear of catheterising was subsiding, and my other responsibilities were getting easier: washing myself, checking my skin for any red marks, tightening the bands on my jaw. Initially, having other people manage my body for me had been welcome, offering me a way to deny reality, but as my strength returned and my understanding of paralysis increased, I wanted to take back control.

And, after five weeks in hospital, I wanted my body *back*.

Thankfully, as it came back into my hands, I noticed that any humiliation about the changes had been relegated to the past. When other people have washed you, changed you, managed your bladder and your bowels for you, and all as nonchalantly as though they were doing it for themselves, embarrassment – like privacy – is forgotten.

In hospital a body just is what it is. There was no shame around the lack of bladder or bowel function. Even as I gradually regained responsibility for my body, it wasn't unusual for the nurses to ask after my bowels in front of my friends or give me a telling-off if I had forgotten to catheterise on time. I welcomed the transparency. It helped me be able to talk openly with my friends. Feeling embarrassed was tiring. Feeling ashamed was *exhausting*.

Having a mum with a nursing background reduced the discomfort even more.

'I started nursing when I was your age, Phie,' she said one day, helping me with a mirror as I fumbled inserting my catheter. 'By your age, I was already clearing up other people's piss, shit and vomit on a daily basis. And as a midwife I've seen it all. You'll get used to it, and at least it's your *own* mess, darling girl.'

Mum had left the nurses' accommodation and moved back home again, but still came almost every day. Past the acute phase of my recovery, my dependency on her had slightly lessened. She had been my protector, speaking on my behalf with the doctors and nurses, helping me care for myself and emotionally supporting me, but I didn't want that to continue. I wished there was more in the manual for how to look after your loved ones, because I so desperately wanted to stop feeling guilty and for her to try and stop worrying about me.

But regardless of the circumstances, spending so much time with her was impacting our relationship for the better. Previously I had only thought of her as a mother; now, I was learning to love her as a woman, and as a friend.

There was one subject, however, that I couldn't bring myself to ask about or discuss with anyone, not even my mum.

Late one night, I had plucked up the courage to venture into the 'Sexual Function' section of the manual. When Emma had mentioned my failing of the 'prick test', all I could think about was if that would also mean an actual *prick*. What solutions were there if that type of test came back negative? Self-catheterising had revealed my body was entirely numb, but what about deep down inside? And what about babies? Had I not been given an answer to this yet? My memory of what I had been told so far was confused by the morphine I had been taking.

But just like every sex education lesson I had ever had in my life, within the manual almost all of the information related to men. The sexual function section focused mostly on how men with spinal injury could get and maintain an erection, and be able to ejaculate.

The only reference to a women's ability to have sex after spinal injury explained that sensation would depend on the type of injury sustained. Through my teary eyes, I didn't find the answer I hoped to. The words *intimacy, pleasure, orgasm* were nowhere to be found.

To me the devastating black hole of information seemed shrouded in shame.

I decided I would just have to forget about sex for the moment. Put it to bed, so to speak, until the time was right.

A friend had given me a book about a man's account of being in a concentration camp in Nazi Germany, in which he wrote that, so long as a person could determine their *why*, they could live any*how*. It was an extreme comparison, but I found it helped. If people could find meaning and purpose in the depths of the worst type of despair, then so could I.

Perhaps I could adapt to all the death in my body, as long as I could find a reason for living.

As the pain in my face decreased, my focus had shifted to the rest of me, but looking in the mirror one morning, I could see that much of the bruising had gone down – stains of yellow marked my face instead of the deep purples and browns of fresh bruises. The stitches, however, had left behind a thin jagged scar that ran down my nose, between my misshapen nostrils, through to my upper lip, which was pulled ever so slightly up by the tightened skin. The bandage had been removed from my eye and the socket was still red and swollen, making my face oddly lopsided. My new nose bent to the left at the top and hooked round to the right at the bottom. Left of my left eye, a purple bruise was surrounded by a pink scar. It was still unnerving to see how I looked but I started to see myself, if not in my features, then in my eyes. I smiled at myself, and the metalwork in my face flashed back. *Goodbye, you fucker,* I thought. It was the day it was being removed.

I recognised Peter Ayliffe as soon as he entered my room. His black hair and friendly face had lingered in my dreams from the moment he'd leant over and winked at me.

'Sophie!' He gave me a squeeze and then hugged Mum. 'Oh look at you, Sophie, haven't you fixed up well!' Muttering to himself as he scanned my face he said, 'Yes, yes, nose is looking good, a little bit wonky but we can fix that eventually. Oh and the eye, yes that's made a good recovery, still a bit bruised – a *lot* bruised, yes – and how about the eye socket? Yes, that's gone down, *great*, as expected. So, now really we just need to get your jaw unwired, don't we?'

With so much going on, I hadn't stopped to consider the discomfort that the procedure might cause me. I'd only just been weaned off morphine. But when you meet the person who helped save your life, you don't want to disappoint them by being a wuss, so I was determined to be brave. But as he started to remove the metalwork, I felt as though he was unscrewing the nerves in my teeth. The familiar raw taste of iron filled my mouth. I closed my eyes and felt the metal releasing. Finally, he stepped back and told me I could open my jaw. The drawer was back on its hinges, and working again. If not a little stiff, but It would loosen up, Peter said. Dribble trickled out of my mouth.

'Oh, don't worry about that,' he said. 'Now look, you might not think that your face looks like it once did, but there's still a bit more recovery yet to happen. I hope the swelling around your eye socket will calm down soon, which will even out your face shape. Your nose has had several bone grafts, the stitches in the area *may* have disturbed it, but we'll see what happens there. Thankfully I had that picture of your face to work from, so I did my best, but I will continue to do so until you're happy, so you must get back in touch with me in the future, whenever you're ready, and we will keep trying to get you back to the girl you once were.'

I gave Peter a slobbery hug and tried to thank him but the words wouldn't formulate properly yet. I just smiled and smiled and smiled. I couldn't stop opening and closing my mouth, like a fish, up and down, up and down. The release was delicious. I hungrily waited for Jack, so I could kiss him, *properly*.

That evening Gary came to see me with a present. 'You've earned it!' he laughed, handing me a packet of cheese and onion crisps. I whooped with delight. 'Gary!' I said, testing how wide my mouth could get. 'You are my HER-OOOOO! Thank you!'

Gary looked at my gums and teeth closely and stepped back. 'Well, Sophie, you seem to be getting back on track.'

As he hoisted me back on to the bed, while I hugged my crisps like a greedy toddler, something caught my eye. I craned around to try to see it. A woman – a vision – in a wheelchair, raced past my room. I could immediately tell from the way she pushed herself that she wasn't like us *newbies;* she was an 'outpatient' so unlike us, she didn't have that vacant confused stare or a dirty brown catheter bag dangling out from the side of her wheelchair. This badass woman had neat cropped blonde hair, and everything about her said, *Do not get in my way*. She looked toned and fit and was also rocking a funky suit, and she had a colourful briefcase on her lap. Her chair was nifty and shiny and moved smoothly over the hospital floor. I begged Gary to hoist me into my chunky old hospital chair so I could follow her but it was too late. She'd shot off into the corridor that led out into the main hospital.

That one glimpse of her was enough to set my imagination into overdrive.

I lay on my bed later that night staring at the ceiling,

chomping jubilantly on more crisps, making up stories about what her life was like, and what her job was, and transplanting myself into them.

Perhaps she was a barrister or a businesswoman.

But did she catheterise? Did she worry about shitting herself in that fancy suit?

What was in her briefcase – catheters and wet wipes?

How did her spinal injury fit into her life?

I was fascinated.

For the first time since the injury, I remembered that I'd wanted to be a lawyer once. I reached under my pillow and scribbled wildly in my diary, doodles of a woman in a wheel-chair with her arms stretched up tall.

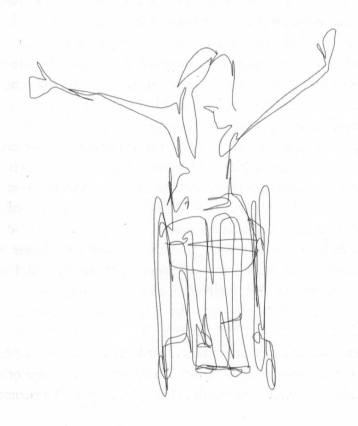

Soph

For the first time in my life, I felt my stubbornness and belligerence could help me. The wayward angst that lay rumbling within me throughout most of my young life now had a target to aim towards and all of my pent-up frustrations became channelled, focused on building a new version of myself.

My consultant gave Gary the go-ahead to move me into the main ward. It was only a matter of metres from the room I had been in for the past six weeks but it felt like a huge move, like going up a year at school, and with the move came extra responsibilities: I would be in charge of getting my own catheters, gloves, 'sups', wipes and incontinence pads each night so that I could manage the mornings. Soon I would be learning how to transfer into my chair without the hoist, and according to the manual, after that it wouldn't be long before I would be able to go home for a visit. The nurses would still oversee my care, but in the ward, more was expected of me; after all, I was two months old, and finally back on solid foods.

I gathered my clutter, took down the cards and photos, and said goodbye to the room, ready to be leaving it and many of the memories it held behind me. I pushed myself down the corridor into the ward where three other women with three other injuries and three other stories were living. They all welcomed me and I smiled back in a way I recalled from the first time I shared a dormitory, open minded to the new people with whom the bookends of my days would be shared. But of course, the commonality between me and the women in the spinal unit was far more significant, as we four shared a traumatic lived experience. As I passed them, I scanned their bodies to see if we had any injuries in common and caught their eyes as they scoured mine. I had seen other in-patients but not up close, and as these were the first people I had really met with spinal cord injury, I wanted to find out how they were. Seeing them in their beds or wheelchairs with the same equipment around them reminded me that I wasn't all alone in this experience. But I didn't let my curiosity get the better of me because the mood in the women's ward was low, none of them were chatty. I was reminded that progress in a spinal unit isn't like progress anywhere else. For most of us, there was no possibility of 'getting better', there was only 'getting out'.

The move into the main ward of the rehabilitation unit meant that my progress could expand, with physiotherapy and OT sessions, one after the other, throughout the day. I brought the manual of doom with me, but packed it away into a cupboard; it was time to put much of what I had read about into practice.

In order to survive in the outside world, I needed to prepare myself for any eventuality. And while I didn't know what to expect, I was pretty sure nowhere would be as accessible as the hospital. With this in mind I asked Debbie and Emma to teach me as much as they could and as I was able to do, and to not allow me to become dependent on any adaptations or unnecessary equipment, unless I absolutely had to. It was time to learn to transfer.

Transfer One was getting on and off the bed into a wheelchair. With no balance, no core strength, relatively little upper-body strength, not to mention being underweight, the effort this required was Herculean. But when I managed to clear the gap and land the leap, the satisfaction levels were off the charts. 'You fucking *go*, girl!' shouted Sara on one of her visits. I couldn't stop laughing. From the disapproving looks on the nurses' faces, I got the impression Sara brought a different kind of energy to that of most visitors – loud and ballsy, instead of frightened and depressed – and I loved it. I needed to be encouraged and then pushed harder.

Transfer Two was the loo transfer, but not just an accessible loo with perfectly positioned grab handles and a heightened seat; I wanted to be able to transfer on to a bog-standard loo so that I could go to the loo at my friends' homes.

Transfer Three involved going from one height to another, the dreaded 'split-transfer', which would enable me to watch TV on a squishy sofa or sit on a barstool.

Transfer Four was getting in and out of the bath. This was my Everest. The effort required to heave myself out of the bath and on to the side was one thing, but sliding on to my chair when slippery wet was another. But I persevered, figuring it would be worth my while as depending on a wet room and shower chair would limit my options moving forward.

The Fifth and Final Transfer was the floor-to-chair move. Emma told me that they didn't typically teach women who were unable to engage their core muscles how to get off the ground into a chair, but nonetheless I gave it my all.

The transfers were like a workout, and I welcomed the sweat. It made me sleep better at night and it distracted me from any unwelcome thoughts. But the past has ways of upending you when you least expect it.

A card had recently arrived from Rory and all that was written were three words: 'Thinking of you'. I had sat looking at them for well over an hour. What did that even mean? I felt unnervingly and unusually needy, desperately searching for

clues in-between the lines, but I found none. I wedged it in my
diary and tried not to think about it again. Thinking about him
felt about as uncomfortable as thinking about *her*, the old me,
the version that walked around in my dreams, and since Jack
had returned and Rory's letter arrived, my dreams had turned
dirty, and waking from them was agonising.

Rehabilitation was the only antidote.

Every successful step I took felt like laying a brick in the road
towards independence.

Day in, day out, I repeated the drills with Emma, occasionally Mum, my friends or Jack, rallying me the whole way. 'You're
the patient all physios dream of, Soph,' she said, and while not
even a specialist Spinal Occupational Therapist would *dream*
of having to teach a completely paralysed eighteen-year-old girl
how to get on and off the toilet again, I understood what she
meant. 'You shouldn't be able to sit up as quickly as you are' and
'You have surprisingly good balance for someone of your level'
felt as good as any chat-up line. 'You're making rapid progress,
Sophie' was about the biggest turn-on I could imagine.

Not what most eighteen-year-old girls might consider a compliment, but for me, the encouragement was just what I needed
to keep going. I could have counted on one hand the number
of times I had been considered a *good girl* in my life. My school
reports read more like crime witness statements, but all that
potential my teachers had hoped I would one day fulfil now felt
achievable. I had an abundance of tenacity in me and, like an
ox, I took on my heavy burden and ploughed on, head down.
(Occasionally shitting as I went.)

Because I still had strength in my arms and hands, a manual
chair would be my best option, as opposed to the larger battery-
powered wheelchairs that I had seen floating around the ward,
controlled with a joystick. But with no 'trunk' muscles, the
back rest would need to be high enough to support me. Emma

found me a chair I could call my own. Heavy and cumbersome, it weighed more than I did and was wide enough for two of me, like wearing a pair of Dad's walking boots, but after she showed me how to push properly, how to turn fluidly, how to go up and down slopes, and how to use the brakes, within no time at all I was chasing Gary around the ward, usually with Boner cheering me on, driving him mad. The smooth floors of the spinal unit were perfect for speeding around, and in time it came close to feeling as liberating as passing my driving test once had.

By far my favourite part of the hospital was the gym. I would sit alone for hours and watch fellow patients as they battled it out with their physios. One of the cruellest drills – the 'catch a ball' drill – was a renowned torture that *sounded* innocent enough but, like waterboarding, was deceptively named. We were made to sit on the edge of a plinth and catch a ball, but with the balance of a drunk, catching a ball with two hands while your back is unsupported is near impossible. I'd watch and laugh sympathetically at other patients who, like me, longed to catch the damn ball and whack their physios over the head with it.

After I got bored of laughing at people, I looked around hoping for any outpatients who might be in for physio. These people fascinated me; the way they transferred so easily and spun their chairs around just as effortlessly was beautiful. Most of the time, I found I was the only female in the gym and while I had read that spinal injury happens to men more than women, it seemed curious. The women I grew up with were every bit as adrenalin-seeking and risk-taking as men. Competing success-fully in a man's world added an extra layer of motivation; seeing young fit men so adapted to their injuries made me want not just to adapt, but to keep up.

*

I had overheard someone talking about weekly basketball training sessions for outpatients and, like a groupie trying to get backstage tickets, I waited by the exit to the gym to catch one of the team to find out when these sessions took place. The following Monday, after I had waved Alick and Jack goodbye, I was there, 8 p.m. sharp, in the front row of the viewing gallery.

A team of wheelchair basketball players was practising in drills that I recognised immediately from all the team sports I had ever played. Every inch of me longed to run in and jump across the court, to intercept one of their long balls, to spin around in mid-air and pass the ball, to be red-hot and sweaty. Seeing these sportsmen throw themselves around the court, their wheelchairs banging and crashing against one another, captivated me. Parts of their bodies looked impaired but there was nothing about them that seemed vulnerable or weak; in fact the complete opposite.

Eavesdropping on their post-game chat, it struck me that there was no mention of the struggles they were having nor of the complexity of their disabilities, they were just like any other team, discussing tactics and gossiping about one another's game. *So*, I thought, *life* does *exist outside of our disabilities, conversations don't have to revolve around what's* wrong *with us*. I wanted what they had. I needed a sport to play.

It was when I discovered that the hospital had an enormous and accessible swimming pool, with a ramp that led down into the water so that specially designed waterproof plastic wheelchairs could roll right into it, I knew that I'd found *exactly* what I was looking for, but when I began to mention this to Emma and others, they told me it would be too soon for someone with my type of injuries. I listened, but to my core, I knew they were wrong.

'Just be patient, princess,' Gary said. 'The time will come.'

Being called 'princess' was beginning to wind me up. Being

told to be patient was grinding me down. I wanted to get out of the cotton wool I was wrapped in. And the insides of the hospital were starting to bore me.

As the weeks turned into months, visitors came to see me less and less, my friends had jobs to do or university to attend. Jack had got a temporary job to support him whilst he continued to live down south, so couldn't visit as regularly as I wished he would, but I didn't mind, I didn't want to be too needy. I had even asked people not to 'waste their time' visiting me. We had all spent years fantasising about all the fun that could be had, free from the rules of school and away from the grasp of our parents, and there was no way I would get in the way of that rite of passage. I didn't want to get in their way, but as the days in rehabilitation blurred into one and the summer turned into autumn, I thought about them all the time, out in the wide world, and wondered what life without interruption, without paralysis, would be like.

Therefore, pushing myself back to my hospital bed one morning, triumphant from a successful practice transfer on to the toilet with Emma – these new metrics for success were so wildly different from those in the life before – I nearly fell out of my chair in shock at the sight of Sophia perched on the end of my bed.

So happy was I to see her, the air left my lungs in an ecstatic gasp. I hadn't realised *just* how much I'd missed her. It had only been about a month since she had started her fresher term, but it felt much more like a year.

'Surprise!' she sang in a mock soprano voice, jumping up and rushing over to me, clamping me close, in a long-overdue hug. 'Surprise, Soph! I'm *so* sorry I haven't been able to visit but honestly, I haven't stopped thinking about you for a moment.'

'Soph! What are you doing here? You are meant to be at uni!'

'I missed you, you twat. I wanted to see how you are! Boner told me you are using a wheelchair now – and look at you. You look *so* much better. Your face has healed up, hasn't it? I heard Jack has come down. How has *that been*? You have to fill me in . . .'

I rolled quickly over to my bed, clicked on my brakes, and as smoothly as I could, transferred over to the bed.

'Holy fuck!' Sophia said. 'Look at you go!'

'I'm getting the hang of it all, Soph, slowly but surely. I tell you, though, it's been hard work.' I didn't want to tell her everything, to go into all the gory details. I didn't want to piss on her parade. There would be another day to share sad stories. That day, I just wanted to hear about her life, the life of a girl unchanged and in her element. I had thought I might feel the sting of jealousy about my friends' stories of freedom, but on seeing Sophia, that doubt had instantly evaporated. Perhaps in the future I was going to have to live more vicariously anyway, so why not start getting used to it? And who better than through my wild and wonderful friend Sophia?

'I don't want to talk about me, I want to hear everything . . .'

For well over an hour, we sat tucked up on my bed together. Her stories carried me up to the wet and dirty streets of Newcastle, where students, set loose, ran amok through the city centre, wearing nothing, caring for nothing, just the next party, the next new friend, the next new album, the next new kiss or shag. She pulled out an iPod and plugged me into the rave music she'd been going out clubbing to, pounding drum and bass climaxing as she bounced up and down on my bed beside me, never for a moment holding back the details she knew I wanted to hear. The fusty stench of nightclub carpets, the clammy feel of two near-naked bodies raving so close together their sweat practically infused, the dread of seeing the sun rise up behind the closed curtain of a hot-boxed student bedroom, the doom of missed lectures or missed phone calls, and the taste of new boys, the fun of new girls, and the temptation of new drugs. She hugged me again, and promised that as soon as I was ready, she would take me with her.

'Soph?' How long Emma had been standing watching us I had no idea, but from the bemused look on her face, I guessed it must have been a few moments. 'Sorry to interrupt, girls, but we have a session now. Time to learn how to "back-wheel balance"!'

'Yes!' I shrieked, the earphone still pumping drum and bass music in my ear.

'What's a back-wheel balance?' Sophia asked as she pulled out the earphones.

'Basically, it's a wheelie,' I said, laughing. 'And I've been waiting for this day for ages.'

Emma smiled. 'It will mean that Sophie will be able to get around a lot easier,' she explained. 'She'll use a wheelie to drop off or jump up kerbs on the street, bounce down steps and stairs, get across uneven ground—'

'Like at a festival?' Sophia cut in.

'Sure, why not?'

'Soph – that is amazing. Let's go . . . Oh wait. Can I come and watch?'

'Of course,' Emma and I said in unison, and in that moment, I felt a brand-new type of happiness. The three of us made our way to the hospital gym, chatting away, and Emma laid out some mats behind me.

'Right,' she said, 'to do this you have to pull your wheels back, as though you're going to go backwards, and then *quickly* flick them forward. This will force your front wheels up, and then you have to balance yourself. You know this is going to be *very* difficult at first, Soph, so don't beat yourself up if you—'

Crash. I had followed her instructions as she had spoken

them but, unaware how hard they would be to follow, I mistimed, unbalanced and slammed straight backwards, cracking
my head on the floor behind me.

'Soph!' yelled Sophia. 'Are you okay?'

There were stars everywhere.

'I wasn't ready to catch you, Sophie,' Emma said, trying to be
sympathetic but clearly irritated. 'You should have waited. For
these first few lessons, I *must* be behind you.'

'I'm fine, Em, sorry, I was over-excited,' I said from the
floor, with my legs in the air and my head throbbing. 'Can you
help me up?'

Sophia was silent, no doubt unsure of what a person is meant
to do when their paralysed best friend falls out of her wheelchair. I smiled at her to reassure her.

'We better get used to this,' I told her. 'I mean, can you
imagine trying to manage one of these when we're drunk!' We
both laughed and it struck me in that moment that every other
laugh we had ever shared had never come close to feeling so
honest, and so helpful.

'Look, girls,' said Emma, a notch less irritated, 'I'll teach you
as much as I can, but just know, there are some things I won't be
able to teach you because you just won't be able to do them . . .'

'Well, that's what I'm here for then, isn't it?' Soph said reso-
lutely, walking around to the back of me to scoop me up and
help return my chair upright.

We spent the rest of the afternoon practising and falling and
laughing. Learning, over and over, how to wheelie, and then
how to wheelie down a step, and then up a step. Sophia got a
spare wheelchair and practised with me, and soon I forgot that
our lives and our struggles weren't the same any more.

Learning how to use a wheelchair came quickly to me. My
hands toughened on the rims of my wheels as I sped around the

hospital corridors and indelible black stains from the dirty tyre treads soon seeped into my skin.

I was realising that people who use wheelchairs are not *wheelchair bound*, not *confined* to their chairs; in fact, this couldn't be further from the truth. We are not bound to them, they are not attached, they are an extension of us and our wheelchairs don't confine us, they liberate us. They carry our bodies when our bodies are unable to carry themselves.

Without our wheelchairs, we wouldn't be able to participate in life.

I also recognised just how much safer I felt with my friend beside me. How, around her, my idea of what might happen to me when I eventually ventured out into the world outside felt slightly less intimidating, and any concerns about the limitations of my body or of my wheelchair lessened at the thought of her being around to pick me up emotionally, as well as physically. Not having to *ask* her to help me closed any gap that I might have imagined between us, and also strengthened and reinforced our connection.

As Sophia waved me goodbye that evening, instead of feeling left behind, I felt as though she left as my foot soldier, my ally, scoping out the world for opportunities that one day, in her company, I may well be able to experience too.

If my chair was to be my chariot, my friends would be the pack to pull and power me forward. Together, surely, we could go anywhere, so long as I held on tight enough.

I thought back to the image of the passive girl in the manual that I had kept in my mind, and gradually, I began to recreate it.

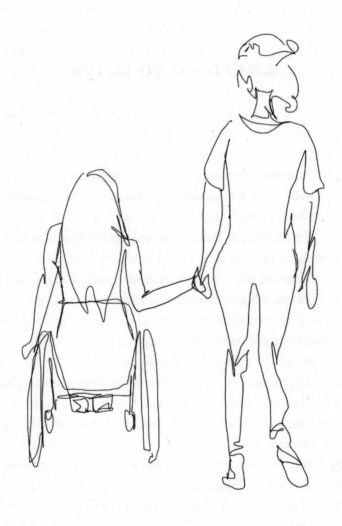

Learning to Drive

One Saturday morning, Dad came screaming into the ward as politely as a man on a mission with the manners of a saint possibly could.

'Mog!' He yelled his lifelong nickname for me. 'You will not *believe* what we've just seen!'

Tom stumbled to a halt behind him. 'Mog!' he echoed. 'You will not believe what we have just *seen!*'

I waited, smiling at them both. 'There's a woman, outside,' continued my dad. 'She's just like you—'

'She's in the car park. She's paralysed too!'

'Soph, she's *driving* . . .' I reached for my wheelchair, clicked on the brakes and transferred across.

'A car, she's driving a car, Mog,' said Tom, practically hopping with excitement.

'She has her wheelchair beside her on the passenger seat!'

'Where?' I said. 'Where is she?!'

'Oh . . .' said my dad. 'She just drove away . . .'

No less than a week later, I was sitting, strapped behind the front wheel of a car, with a local driving instructor who had adapted his car with hand controls. Unable to manage the transfer into a car by myself yet, Dad had lifted me in, and he and my brother stood beside the driver's side of the car watching on, as fascinated and excited as I was. Our delight was infectious, and the instructor broke into a smile just looking at the three of us.

'I take it none of you have seen "hand controls" in a car, then?'

'No, never,' I said.

'We didn't even know they *existed*!' said Dad.

'Okay then,' the instructor said, 'so let me explain. What you've got here is your typical "steering ball" – they help you turn the wheel using just one hand.' The steering ball was attached at the ten o'clock position of the steering wheel. The instructor gave it a twist to demonstrate how it rotated.

'If you look into the footwell, you can see the foot brake and the accelerator of the car – there is no clutch, as this car is an automatic – are attached to a bar, and that to a handle, just on the right of your steering wheel.'

We all craned round to look around the side of the steering wheel and saw a handle about ten centimetres long and about three centimetres wide. I gave it a pull, and sure enough, as I pulled it, the accelerator pedal compressed and when I pushed it, the brake pedal compressed.

'So, seeing as you've already got your driving licence, Sophie, I won't have to teach you much, but driving with hand controls can take a bit of getting used to. It's not complicated or hard, it's just *different*. I usually take drivers out on the quiet roads around the back of the hospital to get to grips with this hand-control system. That sound okay with you?'

'Yes!' I was attempting to bounce up and down, but being unable to, I just flapped my arms. 'Can these two come too?'

I knew they were every bit as excited as I was, so I wanted to share the joy of the moment with them. God knows they had earned some. I hadn't seen my brother in weeks and wanted to show him I was still his big sister, no matter how changed I was. And as my strength was returning, so too was my dad's.

Their shared joy in this pivotal moment felt so sincere to me, it reminded me that these two people meant more to me than ever. They had been shattered by what had happened to me, and we may have lost one another temporarily in the shock, but as we spoke the same language, shared the same values, I knew exactly what that meant: we could find each other again and reconnect in moments like these.

'I think for this first lesson,' said the instructor, 'it's best just the two of us.'

'Yes of course!' Dad tapped on the roof of the car, masking his disappointment well. 'Off you go, guys!' I smiled at them to reassure them both that I would be back safely.

'Next time, though, okay?' I said as I buckled up my seat belt. As I threaded the belt across my chest, I paused. Just where the belt crossed my body was the point where my spine was damaged. *The seat belt may have paralysed me,* I thought, *but it probably also saved my life.*

I clicked in and took the steering wheel in my hands. Breathing slowly and deliberately, I checked around, adjusting my mirrors and making sure it was safe to drive off.

The instructor gave me permission to start the engine. I paused. If there was any time when my fear of driving might have resurfaced, I assumed it would be now, but my hands sat calmly, one on the steering ball and one on the hand control. Tugging the hand-control handle towards me, I eased forward. The weight of the hand control had pulled me forward ever so slightly but pushing my other hand against the steering ball, I counterbalanced.

'Brilliant, that's it!' said the instructor. 'Now, make sure you keep it nice and smooth. Some drivers find the adjustment a little strange, we're so used to using our feet to brake, for example, it can take a little bit of practice till we override that instinct and tell our brain to react using our hand instead. But you will get the hang of it in no time . . . '

He was right. The sensation of driving with my hands was peculiar. Testing the brake, my brain instantly asked my leg to compress the pedal, but the impulse to move didn't bother me; this was not one of those situations in which I yearned to be as I once was. I was still able to drive, even without the use of my legs, and hand controls, a most basic innovation from what I could see, would give me freedom to move and the chance to venture into the world. I was back in the driver's seat and had never felt more ready to get going, to find Ellie and drive in the sunshine with music blaring, fluffy dice dancing.

'This ...' I shouted to the empty road, as we jerked along like a learner testing out their clutch pedal, 'is fucking *EXCELLENT!*'

Back to the Nest

The last time I had been at my parents' home there had been a feeling of change in the air; I was preparing to leave the nest and the summer after I finished school had been a deliriously exciting time, full of newness and those sorts of long August-hot days typically experienced in childhood, with no responsibilities and no worries. And as though I was that little snotty girl in the woods with her dog-friend Sumo, at eighteen my world had revolved around me and my decisions and it was every bit as wonderful as I had hoped it would be. I was on the precipice of the unknown, joyfully oblivious to what was about to happen to my life, looking skyward dreamily and getting ready to take off.

Growing up in a boarding school so far from where we lived meant I didn't feel rooted anywhere in particular, and that's how I liked it. After years of being at school in Scotland, I didn't feel as connected to my parents' house as I once had; it was an address to stop at, between terms, a room to unpack some bags into or a base from which to plot my next getaway.

I had been in rehabilitation for seven weeks, the last month of which I had spent nagging Gary, Emma and whoever would listen, for a dispatch date. I had almost completed all the stages of my education, had just about mastered every transfer and got to grips with the back-wheel balance, and I wanted to have a target to aim towards. I wanted a date to count down to. As ready as I was to leave the hospital, the idea of returning to my parents' house felt like going *backwards*, but it was the only path available to me.

Once again, I felt ready for the next chapter of my life, but no one would consider pinning down a date until our home had been assessed for access.

The morning of my first day visit, I sat on my hospital bed looking at the photograph of me that had been pinned to the wall and took in the background: the garden of our home was where some of my last steps had been taken. Suddenly I worried if I would ever feel at home there again, with my own footprints haunting me?

There was only one way to find out.

I longed to drive myself home, to give me some sense of normality and maturity, but I didn't have an adapted car of my own; instead Mum collected me from the spinal unit and, to avoid over thinking, I slept all the way home in the passenger seat.

'Welcome home!' everyone shouted as Alick carried me out of the car and into the house and plonked me on the kitchen work surface, leaving me feeling as though I might topple off. Instinctively, I tried to jump up and skip off as I once would have done. But I couldn't. Like a sledgehammer, reality hit me. But this was a milestone and there were no tears allowed at milestones (one of my new rules). I smiled sheepishly at everyone and busied myself looking at the floor, fighting back the tears I wished weren't about to bubble over.

Thankfully, Mum got busy tidying up after the dogs; Dad, preparing lunch; Tom was fussing about the music and Alick, who was back from university for the occasion, was helping lay the table for lunch outside in the garden. I wished Jack was there, but he was busy working. He seemed to be working *a lot*.

'What time is Emma getting here?' Dad asked Mum as he

sliced up some tomatoes and poured himself a glass of wine. 'It's a big day, eh, Mog!' he said. I kept my head down and mumbled something like yes.

The same rigmarole and protocols for a dinner party were being applied, the same wine glasses and table decorations being arranged, and the same music was playing. It was dizzying. Perched on the work surface, I tried my hardest not to keep thinking about standing up. With nowhere else to look but at my thin, toneless legs, which dangled over the side, and the Ugg boots on my unresponsive feet, I couldn't get the thought out of my mind. I willed myself to stand. Nothing. *Wake up*, I screamed inside. Nothing. A teardrop landed on my thigh. Quickly I rushed to wipe it away, but in the kerfuffle around me, no one noticed anyway. And then the cascade started and I watched as tears patted down on to my grey tracksuit bottoms.

'Well, we left an hour before her,' said Mum, oblivious. 'So hopefully she shouldn't be that much longer.'

'So,' said Dad, 'the plan is to have some lunch, and then what, you show her around the house?'

'We're going to have to decide which parts of the house need adapting,' said Mum, still too busy to notice, 'which room will be the best for Phie, and generally just have a good chit-chat about how to make the cottage as accessible as possible.'

I'd never known how lonely and invisible it is possible to feel in a room full of people you love. *I wasn't meant to be here; I had left this nest.* I wiped away the tears on my sleeve and held up my face to smile at everyone.

'Can I do anything to help?' I asked.

Everybody stopped and looked at me as though they'd just noticed I was still there.

'Don't be *silly!*'

'You just sit there, and we'll get everything ready.'

There was no point asking for my wheelchair as the house

was filled with stairs. I'd never noticed how many there were before – I could see four steps just to get from the kitchen out to the garden. The doorways seemed narrower than I'd ever noticed before. *And since when were the floorboards so uneven?* The house was not as I remembered, *no*, it was *I* who was not as I remembered. I felt disorientated, and the more familiar it all was the more removed I felt.

Away from the hospital, I had a sinking feeling that the sense of not belonging might pervade.

I returned to watching my legs, silently praying that being home might wake them up. *People talk about muscle memory, so maybe being in the house, in this memory, they could be reminded they used to work?*

No response.

The line remained dead.

'Mum,' I said, as I realised I wouldn't be able to get into the downstairs loo in my wheelchair, 'I'm gonna need to catheterise in about fifteen or twenty minutes ...?'

'I've already thought about that,' she said. 'The sitting room. I got all the extra stuff from Gary. Tom, would you mind helping Phie?'

I was somewhere between grateful and utterly distraught at the thought of my brother helping me to the loo, and whatever that internal chaos did to my face must have been telling, as Tom approached me apprehensively, his eyebrows high, his arms outstretched. On the one hand, I was appreciative of the love and support that I was getting, but on the other hand, the idea that I could no longer go to the loo by myself, that I wasn't able to help myself, or help them, made me want to burn the whole goddamn house to the ground. I was boiling with fury and at the same time overflowing with gratitude.

'Want a lift next door?'

Worried that if I opened my mouth, something toxic would

come out, I just pacified the situation with a smile and a nod and let him pick me up off the work surface.

'I never thought about how small the loo was. Did you?' Tom said as he carried me up some stairs and through a crooked wooden door into the sitting room, placing me gently down on to an armchair. Mum followed behind him carrying catheters, a bottle, an incontinence pad, wet wipes and hand sanitiser and put them down on the armchair beside me, along with a mirror. I stared blankly at all this. It belonged in the hospital, not in our cosy, comfy cottage in the forest.

'Do you want help,' asked Mum, 'or are you going to be all right to do this by yourself?'

'No, no. I'm fine. I've had a lot of practice and I'm getting better,' I said. This wasn't absolutely the truth, but I needed some time alone.

With the door closed, I pulled down my tracksuit bottoms and started to catheterise, but sitting in the armchair with no proper back support, I lost my balance. Toppling over I dropped everything, and it all clattered on to the floor. I straightened up and got a fresh catheter. I tried to hold the mirror in front of me to help me see, but I didn't have enough room to rest it securely and it fell to the floor. I recovered the mirror but in all of the mess and fuss, it was too late, and I hadn't got the incontinence pad underneath me. There was urine all over the armchair.

I was about to sink further into despair, but in that mortifying moment something held me back. I picked up the wet wipes, tidied myself up, wiped my face, blew my new nose and then dropped down on to the floor so that I could assess the damage on the armchair. A dark wet patch across the seat of the white armchair. I pulled off my T-shirt and started dabbing away at the mess, trying to dry the stain. Cleaning up my own mess felt good. In fact, doing anything to help myself felt good. I pressed harder, and slowly the T-shirt started to soak up the mess.

'MUM,' I shouted. 'Please can you get me a new pair of pants, a T-shirt and trousers and bring down a towel?!'

I heard a clatter of footsteps as Mum rushed into the sitting room.

'Why? What's happened? Are you okay? What's ... oh!' She saw the stain.

'I'm so sorry, I made a right mess—'

'Oh for crying out loud, who gives a flying fuck? It's just a chair. It's just *wee*. It's like puppy piddle, as far as I am concerned. No point crying over spilt ... piss ...'

The two of us burst out laughing and she gave me a hug.

'Let's get you cleaned up. Emma will be here in a minute and we don't want her to see you lying on the floor half undressed. She won't ever let you come back home again.' Mum flipped the armchair cushion and collected up the rubbish. 'The only reason they allowed us to have this home visit so early on is because I promised I'd look after you.'

'Right then.' I started to strip off my wet clothes and get changed. 'Let's not let her down.'

Eventually Emma arrived and we all sat together in the garden, in the sunshine. Dad passed around his homemade spaghetti Bolognese and topped up wine glasses. Tom and Alick played with the puppy. The old dog slept under the table. *The dogs,* I thought thankfully, *don't see me as any different. They have no idea what's going on.* Music drifted over from an open window. If you didn't know what this meeting was about, it would have looked fun.

But I was torn between my two clashing worlds: my parents in their roles of host and hostess, over lunch with my occupational therapist, whose purpose it was to redesign their home for their newly paralysed daughter. It felt both comforting and horrifying.

In preparation for this very conversation, Emma and I had

discussed the types of adaptations that I might need at home, and I'd been very clear that wherever I could, I wanted to avoid permanent and complicated adaptations. It was important to me that I adapted to the world, and not the other way round. Emma knew this about me, it had been a point of contention to begin with, but over time she could see that I was so determined, it was best, where possible, to let me get my way. Still, regardless of what I wanted, as the cottage was over two floors, I would need a lift to get upstairs, and with steps throughout the house, ramps would need to be put down.

As a feeling of depression crept over me, I tried to remind myself that these adaptations would enable me to come home and live independently and that was all that mattered. I may have wanted to leave the nest, but circumstances meant I had to return, and the fact my family were adapting it for me was about the greatest possible testament of their love. *Don't be a brat*, I told myself, as I watched Mum and Emma walk into the house and disappear upstairs, and resisted the urge to shout up at them that I wanted to join in and that these were my needs they were assessing. Yes, people would go places I could no longer get to; they would have conversations on my behalf without me; I would have to amend my expectations. *Be grateful for what you have.* I was going to have to adapt my mentality every bit as much as I would have to adapt my home, I told myself.

'How long do you think till I get used to this, Dad?' I asked, watching Emma through one of the upstairs windows. The question was rhetorical. I could have been asking about any of it or all of it – my paralysis, my wheelchair, my mother making decisions about my life, the adaptations in our home, adaptations to our lifestyle. And how could he answer anyway? How could anybody know how long it would take for me to adapt to the situation? That was entirely up to me.

But I asked anyway because it stopped me from freaking out.

Dad topped up my wine glass and moved back in his chair. The early autumn sun hit his hair and it looked bleached and blond once more. 'Just take one day at a time, and where there are problems,' he said, his blue eyes shining, 'let's work together as a family to find solutions. Because that's what we do.' He took a big glug of wine and smiled. '*That's* the Morgan Way.'

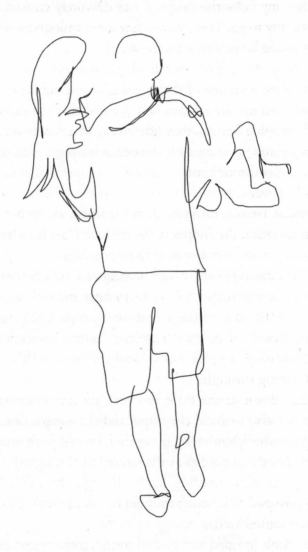

When I returned to the spinal unit, pushing myself around the hospital corridors reminded me of those restless final days of school. I felt I had outgrown it. I was getting bored of the women I shared a ward with, irritated with the endless alarms ringing, tired of being called princess and fed up of waiting. I knew all the nurses and hospital staff by name, the hospital café even knew my favourite crisps. I was definitely cooked. But I still had a way to go. There were a few more milestones to reach before I would be permitted to leave.

Bone came down from Scotland one weekend, and I asked her to help me with one of them: going out in public.

We weighed up our options and decided that as much as we disliked shopping centres, they offered my wheelchair as accessible an environment as possible outside of hospital, with smooth floors and lifts throughout.

So, off we went.

But about twenty minutes in we realised we hadn't taken into consideration the shoppers themselves. Dawdling and distracted, they made moving next to impossible.

'I've tried asking politely, but no matter how many "excuse me"s I might say, they don't seem to hear me unless I shout EXCUSE ME!' Bone yelled and the crowd scattered, like pigeons escaping a dog. My wheelchair charged into them, only narrowly missing people's ankles and the toes of their shoes. '*Move*! Coming through . . .'

I looked down at the floor to check for any potential trip hazards, but also to avoid the stares and the gawps. Boner was pushing my wheelchair much faster than I could push myself, so I kept my hands on my lap as she steered us through the many shoppers that were ambling lazily through the mall. 'These fucking *peep-pul*! Why don't they get out of the way? EXCUSE ME!' she shouted louder.

More people jumped and turned round, some tutted angrily,

some apologised and stared. Boner laughed. 'Thank you,' she said sarcastically.

We were in Tunbridge Wells; the very same stomping ground I'd once terrorised as a young teenager I now rolled over as a wheelchair user. Where once young boys would have turned to look at me, maybe given me a cheeky wink, or even catcalled, now there was nothing but curious, nosy, sideways glances, or outright unapologetic stares and affronted tuts. Never one to care about people staring at her, I could tell Boner wasn't bothered by the spectacle. Yet I, feeling so unseen and yet so stared at, was slightly disconnected.

I started looking up and holding my head a little higher.

'Oi! Watch where you are going!' a middle-aged woman shouted at us, as Boner skimmed past her and my shoulder knocked her shopping bag. I could tell Boner was running as she pushed me; between shouts she was slightly out of breath and panting. We were rushing to get out; the claustrophobia was getting to us both. We were better suited to being in the woods together, not a city-centre shopping mall.

I tried to spin round to gesture an apology, but Boner swerved and kept going.

'People are so *rude!*' My friend shouted this loudly over her shoulder so the woman would hear, but also for my benefit. It made me smile. A nice healthy dose of hypocrisy. But she had a point: who was being ruder? Us ploughing through the crowds as though we had right of way or the many people who stopped and stared as I rolled past?

Some little kids pointed at me. 'Mummy, Mummy, what's wrong with that girl?' They tugged on their mum's jeans and she hushed them quickly, then gave me a nod as though to apologise on their behalf. A group of boys, not much older than my brother, stopped to stare; one of them pointed at the wheelchair and laughed. Two young girls, not too dissimilar from

Bone and me, were slurping on their drinks, their hands full of handbags and shopping bags. One turned to the other and said, 'She's quite pretty for a wheelchair, isn't she?' The friend replied, 'Yeah ... it's a shame, isn't it?' A middle-aged woman caught my eye and tilted her head sympathetically to one side. An old man observed my wheelchair and joked to us, he would need 'one of those' soon.

'Excuse me,' I found my voice. A family who had been ambling in front of us spun around, the mum snatched up her child rapidly. 'Get out of the way,' she shouted at the child, who broke out in tears and looked at me, terrified.

I wasn't sure who was more scared: him of me or me of the situation.

Bone may have been pushing my wheelchair through the crowds like a battering ram, but I was thankful, because the words and looks coming at me felt like an assault. She kept pushing me, searching for the exit, trying to escape. We finally made it through the glass double doors, relieved for the fresh air. The rain splattered down but we weren't bothered. Boner released the back of my chair and ran ahead to look for some cover. We ducked under a shop awning and stopped to roll some cigarettes.

'Well, that was a *mission*. You're definitely going to need to use that voice of yours, Morgan.'

'I know, it's just *so* hard; they don't seem to see me ...'

'I guess it's because you're so low down now. You're going to need thick skin, aren't you?'

'Boner, *you* are like armour for me. Honestly, it would be so scary without you. I would feel so defenceless, and so small!'

'As small as Ellie?' We laughed.

'You know what I mean, though? To go from five foot nine to what? Four foot? It's fucked. It's a whole new perspective. Everyone keeps staring at me. I just want to fit in—'

'No, you don't, Sophie Morgan. You have never wanted to fit in. And if you start, well, then we're through.' Boner winked at me.

I smiled at my friend, thinking back to when we first met, and knew that as long as I had her, and the others, half of this extraordinary battle was already won.

I was eighteen years old and I was two months old, and the world was starting to open up again. Thoughts of the future had returned, although only vaguely. But it wasn't as straightforward as I hoped it would be. Thinking about what was next, it became obvious that whatever used to drive me forwards was no longer the same. My motivations weren't altogether clear, but whatever was next had to be well considered.

You don't die once, I wrote in my diary, *not to make the most out of living twice.*

Can You Feel It?

E mma had pointed out that my old bedroom in the cottage had too many steps leading into it, so for my first overnight visit a week later, I had been put in the spare room. Lying on my back in bed with the lights slightly dimmed, I realised that I had never slept in that room before, I didn't recognise the curtains. But, I checked myself, I shouldn't be thinking about the curtains.

The time had come to put my body to the test.

When Jack climbed into bed beside me, the routine of move-ments we knew so intimately started out as normal. Helping one another, we peeled our clothes off slowly; he held my back for balance, I undid his belt. He lifted me and I positioned myself, and apart from the scars and the softness of me, he said he couldn't notice any difference. I wanted to believe him, but I didn't; it didn't matter what I believed, what mattered was that to him, *she* still existed. We kissed the same as we always had, except it felt more generous than before, maybe even more tender. I held his head closer than I remember ever doing before and then guided his mouth to the side of my neck then around to the hollow between my collarbone, where I released him, and watched as he kissed and stroked my chest. Before he went any further, he came back to my face and I nodded permission to go ahead. His hands disappeared beneath the invisible level of my paralysis, and I held my breath in hope, but when he manoeuvred himself between my legs and asked me if I could feel it, I knew in an instant that my life would never be the same again.

'Can you feel it?' He whispered kindly. 'Can you feel it, Soph?' My body moved in rhythm with his. His breath against my face.

I watched as he moved himself inside and out of my body, and I may as well have been watching someone else. I felt suffocated and disorientated. But worse than that, I felt absolutely nothing.

'Yeah,' I lied. 'It feels good. Keep going.' He wanted me to be happy as much as I wanted him to be happy, so I lied because he sounded so hopeful, and I didn't want to let him down. My body didn't hurt, and watching him enjoy me felt as good as anything I had experienced so far, so I lied to him because I didn't want him to stop. He moved my body, lifted my hips and enjoyed me as he always had. I touched my breasts and closed my eyes and for a split second, my mind pretended it was satisfied, but I wasn't. I opened my eyes and looked away. To him everything must have looked and felt the same; for me, the curtains were still unrecognisable.

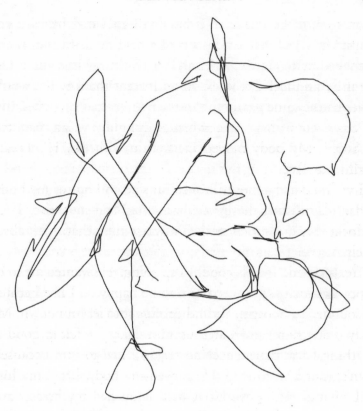

The following morning I came down the wooden ramp that had been nailed into the kitchen floor, to a room full of welcomes from my family.

'Morning, Mog!' said Dad. 'Did you sleep okay?'

I so desperately wanted to say 'no', but the word appeared to have been wiped from my vocabulary. Even though it tottered on the tip of my tongue, I hadn't been able to say it. Not to Jack, and now not to them. *No* just felt too negative and we had no more time for the negatives; coming home was meant to be a positive step. *No sad tears on milestones, remember.*

If I had been honest with them all then I would have told them that, no, I did *not* sleep okay. Because *no*, it turns out my

worst fears had come true. I couldn't feel it and after I faked
a finish and Jack fell asleep, with his arm draped lovingly but
numbly over my stomach and his face nestled against mine, I lay
in the dark and tried to work out what life without feeling would
be like. The vague paragraph in the manual had suggested that
for some women with spinal cord injury there was a chance of
sensation, and deep down I'd hoped that, *deep deep down*, I
would feel something. But in the act, the truth had been handed
to me, and it had not only broken my already fragmented heart,
it had also turned me into a liar. I had had my reasons. I'd
thought they made sense at the time, but in the cold light of day,
I wasn't sure. Yet as pity had only *just* started to leave the faces
of those around me, I thought that perhaps sometimes it's just
easier to pretend, to fake your own happiness – in bed and in
life – than it is to open up and confess that really, *no*. No, you
really feel nothing at all or no, you really are not okay.

So early that morning, lying beside the one person who had
loved me and loved my body – possibly even more than I ever
had – I had tried to work out whether or not my memories of
us having sex together would sustain me, or if they would haunt
me. I had lain in the dark wondering if it was better to know
how it felt to be tickled on the inside of your thigh, to be kissed
on your belly or licked into orgasm by another's mouth? *And
what about knowing what it feels like to run? To hide? To seek?
To walk in high heels?* Is it better to have tasted the tantalisingly
moreish slice of adult freedom I had had for two months, or
eight weeks, or fifty-six whole days, or is it *not*? *Is my life going
to be filled with comparison?*

In the dark, I had decided I couldn't ever know, but whatever
the truth, some of my favourite and now most treasured memories were shared with the person lying next to me. He too had
memories of my body: the positions it could be in, the shape it
cut, the pleasure it gave and the way it moved. So maybe I could

leave my body, *her* body, to him in memory, to keep safe in case one day, I might forget what I was once like.

I had thought with a jolt that there was a possibility that this boy had given my young body the most pleasure it would ever know. That I might never orgasm again.

But I didn't *want* to believe it wasn't possible to find pleasure, there must be other ways. Sex could be about more than penetration, couldn't it? Disabled people *must* have sex? My sex drive was still the same, maybe the act of sex could adapt? Maybe one day I could find someone else who could help me find out what was possible in all the seemingly impossible. It was too hard to imagine doing this with Jack. He loved the other me, and I didn't want to ask him to try to love this new me. What if he said he couldn't?

I had kissed him on the forehead as he slept and knew that I would have to leave him where I loved him . . . in the past.

He'd told me that week that he had plans to be in the mountains soon, and so it would be best to let him go anyway, especially as I had no idea how I could ever follow him there.

The thought of him leaving made me fretful, but if anything, perhaps it meant I was back where I started, ready to move out into the world, by myself. Although our chapter had been temporarily reopened, and I would forever be grateful, maybe it was time to close it again. Time to meet new people, make new connections.

And it was that thread of hope that had eventually pulled me into sleep.

But hours later, when I was asked how I was, I said none of these things.

Instead, I pushed myself across the kitchen over towards the dogs, and transferred on to the sofa to cuddle up to old Sumo, her hair still the same colour as mine, and I pushed my face into hers, and breathed in the smell of the past, and instead of breaking down, I gave thanks because, I looked around me, Dad had got the twinkle in his eyes back. Mum had stopped smoking. Tom wasn't pinching his skin raw any more. My friends hadn't left me behind. There were good, kind people in my life, new emotions to experience, wine to drink and music to dance to and friends to laugh with and, I squeezed her tight, dogs to hug. I was still alive and there were reasons to be happy *still*, reasons to *live*, and who knows, one day, maybe great sex could happen again.

So, instead, I smiled and said, 'Yes, I slept fine, thank you. And it is so good to be back.'

Miracle Man

For all I had been told about my spinal cord injury, the defiant part of me didn't always take it as fact. Just as I had harboured hope that I might still feel sex, I concealed another desperate desire: that perhaps someone, somehow, could be wrong and that maybe, just maybe, there had been a mistake and that I could be one of those stories, those ones you see about the person who 'defied the odds', 'proved their doctors wrong'.

I'd even imagined a grainy photograph of my family and I standing up together, hugging, under a headline that read 'The Girl Who Didn't Give Up'.

I didn't give voice to this wish, burying it, but over two months since my injury, like a cancer it had spread and toxic thoughts of denial had proliferated into the corners of every part of my mind.

It wasn't until a newspaper arrived on my bed, followed by Mum grinning maniacally, that I recognised the same malcontent existed in her too.

'Have a look at this article, Phie. This girl was just like you and she's taken some steps!' She tapped the paper so forcefully my hospital bed rattled. A young woman who had sustained a complete spinal injury in an auto accident was walking again.

I looked up at Mum. She smiled at me. 'Read it all . . .'

The article explained that the young woman was able to 'initiate movement in much of her body below the injury site for the first time since injury, including standing and taking up to 20 steps thanks to a miracle worker called Hratch Ogali'.

I read the article once, and then read it again.

Although Mum and I had never divulged our desires for a cure, I wasn't at all surprised she shared the same hope as I did. As a woman adept at fixing problems, the hopelessness of my spinal cord injury must have cut her more deeply than she cared to admit.

I looked back over the article again. It was heaving with words like 'determination' and 'courage'. It told us how the young woman 'refused to give up' and suggested that it was the power of positive thinking that had saved her.

'You need to have determination and never give up,' she told the reporter, 'I hope I can show other people with similar problems what can be achieved.' The article then focused on Hratch Ogali, who claimed that by simply talking to patients and getting them to focus on inactive muscles, he could help them regain movement. A former jeweller, he now called himself a 'mind instructor'.

I had never understood science as a girl, but I did know a thing or two about breaking the rules. I knew about throwing all my energy at something till it broke. I knew about anger, and fighting. I knew about will-power.

'If anyone has determination, Phie, it's you.' Mum sat beside me and we looked at the photo of the young woman. I needed to see this miracle worker. We called the number in the article. Hratch Ogali could see me, but I would have to wait a few weeks. I buried the article in my diary, and waited, distracting myself with rehab once more, but internally a stopwatch had started and with it, the race to my escape. Maybe I wouldn't have to deal with this for much longer.

Two weeks later, I was on my way in a specially adapted taxi to central London to see the miracle man. There was no good luck or fingers crossed as I left the ward with my parents. Gary had refused even to talk to me about it and my consultant, Emma and Debbie advised us all this was a dangerous and futile endeavour. But Mum and I had read the article, and we had to know for ourselves; if there was a cure, we would get it. There was no going back.

A few hours later, the personalised number plate OGALI on the spotless cream Bentley confirmed we had found the address, and we were ushered through into the Revolution International Clinic.

Hratch Ogali walked into the room and took a seat in the large rotating armchair behind his wide wooden desk, exuding the confidence of a man who had the words 'Mind Instructor' carved into a plaque on the wall above him. His white linen shirt, so crisp it raised up as he sat, protruded from his stomach like a bib. Gold rings squeezed on to his fingers, and a matching-coloured chain winked at me from around his drooping neck.

'Hello, young lady,' he said, swivelling his chair as he looked me over. 'I understand that you have a spinal cord injury sustained in an automobile accident. Let me see my notes here, August the eighteenth, and you saw my recent article, yes?' He had a clipped accent that sounded Arabic or Turkish to me.

'Yes, it was amazing. Mum and I are so intrigued . . .'

'What date is your birthday?'

'Excuse me?'

'Your birthday, when were you born?'

'Oh, um, in February 1985, I'm nineteen in about four months' time, on the twenty-fourth . . .'

At my answer he heaved himself out of his chair, which gave a puff of relief as it repositioned, and rushed straight towards me, placed his forefinger in-between my breasts, pressed me firmly and declared with eyes closed that yes, I would definitely walk again.

With these words still reverberating around the room, he returned to his throne and pulled out a leather planner to check when exactly my Miracle could fit into his diary. A time and date were agreed, and we were corralled out through the door, but not before he crouched down in front of me, took one of my feet, and told me to try to move my leg. Baffled but steadfast, I closed my eyes and imagined moving my leg. I couldn't see where his hands were but suddenly my leg jumped.

I looked at Mum. Her mouth was slung open like a brown paper bag for hyperventilating. She had witnessed it.

'*You* just made your leg *move*,' he said.

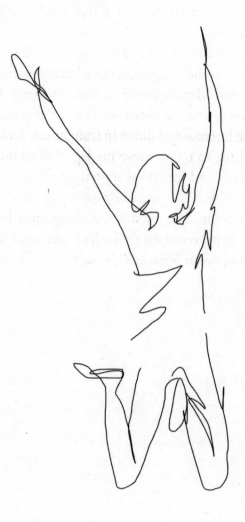

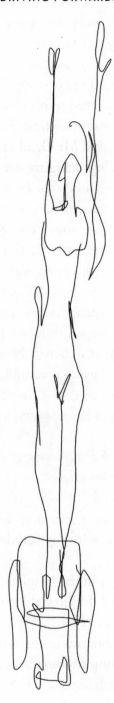

I kept the prognosis secret from my team. They didn't ask questions because they didn't believe in him and I wanted to prove them wrong, so I carried on with my rehabilitation as usual, but eagerly awaited my first appointment.

A few days later I returned to his clinic.

A plinth exactly the same height as Emma's in the gym sat in the centre of the room, and Mr Ogali instructed me to transfer on to it, and leave my legs hanging over the side. He raised it up so that my feet didn't touch the floor.

'Now, what I want you to do is visualise energy running through your spine. Close your eyes, go into your brain and down the spinal cord and activate all the nerve endings that were connected before the cord was severed.' I wanted to correct him because my spine wasn't severed exactly, just damaged, but he continued, 'Allow that energy to flow and focus as deeply as you can on different parts of the body until you feel them.' I did as instructed. Nothing happened. 'This will take time, Sarah.' Again, I wanted to correct him, but he kept talking. 'This session is the first of many, and you will need to continue this exercise every night before you go to bed, okay?'

I closed my eyes, thought about the young woman walking in the article, and gave him a nod.

'Of course, yes, I can do that. Thank you.'

The session lasted an hour, and while no progress was made, I felt assured that with my full dedication I would soon see results.

After that, every night in the hospital (or on my visits home), just before I went to bed, I followed his instructions. Mr Ogali had told me that unless I truly believed in his method it wouldn't work, so, I put any scepticism out of my mind and meditated on his dogma: visualising my breath carrying healing powers into my spine and dissolving the scar tissue that was blocking it. I pictured the girl I once was, captive within me, waking up. I pictured her running off to my command. I imagined her strutting, dancing, running, fucking.

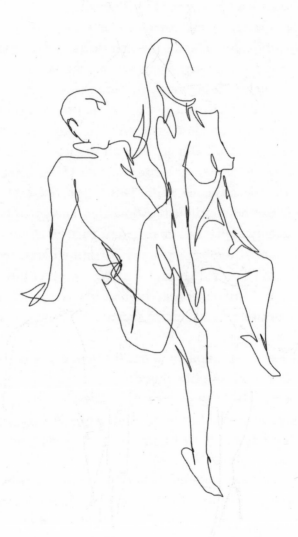

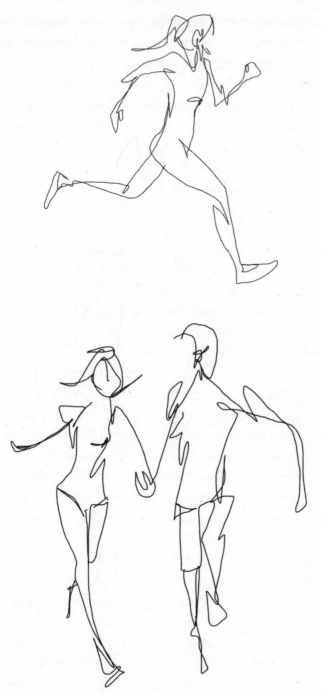

I sat on the side of my bed, fixed my eyes on my paralysed feet as they hung limp, and concentrated with an intensity on which my life depended. I directed everything inwardly, all my energy, straining so hard the veins in my neck pounded, and sweat beads trickled down on to my clenched jaw.

Each night I would collapse, like a marathon runner whose body couldn't withstand the distance, battered and defeated, yet still certain that the next night would be the one, that I just needed to believe a little harder. Like a devout monk, flagellating myself over and over and over, every night I tried to make my legs move.

I wrapped up my dream like a precious Christmas present, and kept it to myself, waiting for the moment when I could bound up off my bed and into my family's arms. I imagined I would shout, *Surprise!* And that Mum would collapse again, but this time I would be there, able to catch her.

I even took his article out of my diary, and pinned it to my wall like a vision board, and underneath the headline I tacked one of the last photographs taken of me standing.

Mr Ogali had suggested that as soon as I was discharged from the hospital, I should move to be closer to his clinic. Apparently, if I really stood any chance of recovery it would take more dedication, more time and much more money. This, he insisted, was our only solution. Mum and Dad assured me the latter was not an issue – 'we can always sell the house' they said.

The hospital knew what I was doing but had long since given up on advising me to stop. I was full of hope and expectation and there was no room for doubt, I told them. Despite their feelings about this 'charlatan', the team were pushing forward with their mission to get me home, equipping me with the skills I would need to live in the world as a paraplegic. They could tell I wasn't as engaged as usual, that I thought their efforts were going to be wasted because any minute now, *just you guys wait*, any minute now I would be fixed.

But no matter how many standing-up hugs I visualised late into the night, I just couldn't seem to make my legs move. I didn't dare admit to anyone just how terrified I was that I didn't quite know how to find the sheer amount of determination that seemed to be required.

Finding me lying despondent on my bed, deflated from yet another failed session at the central London clinic one after-noon, Emma tried to rally me with some good news.

'Guess what, Soph? We have a dispatch date for you!'

I didn't respond.

Emma asked me to sit up and swing my legs over the side of my bed.

'Well, you've certainly got the hang of that manoeuvre, hav-en't you? Look how easily you pulled yourself up and here you are, sitting up straight with good posture despite not having *any* core, holding yourself up so well. I am proud of you, well done you,' she said, satisfied with her work.

'I didn't tell you about it because I know you think it's all mumbo-jumbo and that I am just a gullible fool, but the mind instructor has given me similar exercises to do every night before I go to sleep. His start in exactly the same way, Em.'

'What does he ask you to do next, Soph?'

'I have to visualise my feet moving . . .'

'And then what?'

'Then they move . . .'

'Have they moved yet, honey?'

'Not yet, but I just have to try harder.'

Crouching down, Emma went quiet. She reached to get my trainers. One of her hands took hold of my dangling leg and guided my foot into the shoe. Suddenly my leg jumped.

'Em! Look! I just did it!'

The thrill nearly knocked me off balance. Finally, my hard work had paid off in front of the one audience I longed to impress. Shocked, Emma looked up at me, her face completely perplexed.

'What did you do?'

'It jumped, my leg, I made it move. IT MOOOOVED!'

The expression on her face contorted, furrow lines clustered in-between her eyebrows.

'Look, watch, Em. I'll do it again, wait . . . ' I strained, closing my eyes and readying myself with a deep breath just as I had been shown. I tried again, thrilled to have the chance to prove Em wrong. I let all the smiling faces of my friends back into my mind as I focused. *Surprise!* I shouted inside. *Jump, for fuck's sake, leg – move!*

Nothing.

'Em, just wait a min, I had it.'

Emma asked me to stop trying. She told me to open my eyes. She ran her fingertips under the soles of my feet and, just like that, my leg jumped in the exact same way it had with Mr Ogali.

'Look.' She did it again. 'It's an involuntary spasm, lovey. If you tickle under your feet, sometimes they jump. It's not *you* moving it, love, it's like a reflex. You know that, you read about them, you have had spasms, haven't you?'

Emma looked at me with a softness I hadn't seen in her before. It made my eyes fill with tears instantly. To prove her point, she tickled the underneath of my foot and my leg jumped again.

'But . . . ' The tears trickled out of me. 'But . . . he said . . . he said *I* made it move . . . and he helped that other woman walk, Em. She had a spinal injury, and she *walked*.'

'Maybe she was an *incomplete* injury and she responded to his physiotherapy? Does this man understand you have a very different one, that a complete injury like yours is different?'

Emma reached in to hug me. 'But, he said . . . it . . . would . . .

work ... I believed ... he said I moved it voluntarily ... Maybe it will?'

Emma hugged me harder and I felt all of the hope squeezed out of me.

'Sophie, we have a discharge date. You've come so far, darling. You have so much life to live. Please don't give all your energy to something that might never happen. Look how upset you are ...'

But he had told me I would walk and I'd believed him. What a fool I felt. What upset me most was that in order for his performance to work, I had invited myself on to his stage willingly, as an accomplice; I had urged him on, complicit in his deception in order for there to be the slightest chance that the trick would work. Had I fallen for the cruellest practical joke imaginable?

I was devastated. But my devastation quickly morphed into outrage.

'How *could* he, Em?' I wiped up my tears and let go of her. 'He told me I would walk, that all I had to do was to *believe* in him. He was in the papers and ... and ... that girl ... she said you just need determination. The fuckers. The fuck-er. I could kill him. In fact, I might paralyse *him*.' My sobs turned into giggles. Morbid giggles of revenge. 'See what he does then, the evil conniving manipulative bastard.'

'You know, I could tell you "I told you so", but I have a feeling you might—'

'Oh don't you dare! I mean, you *should*, but don't you dare.' I laughed and took a deep cleansing breath. 'So that's it. This is it.' I tried not to cry ... 'It's never going to go away, is it, Em?'

'Well, never say never, but ... there might be a cure one day.'

'Cure ...' I repeated the word ruefully. '*Cured*.' It didn't sound to me like a relief or a restoration any more, it reminded me of meat, cured meat, preserved through manipulation. An act by a person to maintain a thing to their own taste.

I looked at Emma, the spinal unit around me, and thought about my family and support network, and realised how problematic it could be if I were to spend more time trying to fix my paralysis than learn how to live with it instead. Perhaps one day there would be a cure, a medical intervention that might help me walk again or, at the very least, feel parts of my body again, but if I were to dedicate my time to finding one, would I miss out on my chances of adapting to the situation as I was? Would I live this life wishing to always be the person I was before, instead of coming to terms with the person I was to be now? It made me wonder about how many other people like me had suffered as collateral damage in the eyes and hands of those who believe that we need fixing. But maybe it's not *us* that need fixing, but the belief that we need fixing that needs fixing.

I signalled for Emma to get my wheelchair and transferred across, the swoop was now quick and effortless.

Suddenly I remembered. 'Wait – did you say something about a *dispatch* date, Em?'

Emma walked purposefully beside me, like an owner proudly showing off her pet, and I loved her for it.

'Yes, Soph, you will be going home in three weeks' time.'

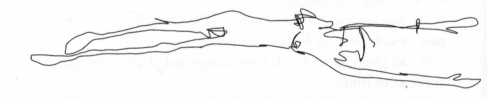

Learning to Swim

B efore I knew it, it was only a matter of days before I would be free, and in anticipation, I had already started to pack. One afternoon I was sitting on my bed, waiting for Gary to sign off my work. Gary came and sat beside me, I handed him the folder, and I watched him thumb through my answers.

Looking over his shoulder, the section on the bladder no longer looked so disturbing, and the bowel management section all made sense. Learning about the respiratory system had taken a while but I had picked up the relevant information and knew my cough was compromised and what to do about it. Some sections didn't relate to my level of spinal injury, so I had skimmed over sections to do with 'autonomic dysreflexia', and spent much more time reading about skin management and how to look after my body temperature.

It had given me so much information and yet, so very little at the same time.

'My work here is done,' Gary laughed, snapping the folder closed. 'How are you feeling about going home then, princess?'

'To tell you the truth, Gary, right now, I don't fucking know. I have dreamt about being 'free' for years, long before my injury, and you know I have been gagging to get out of here since I arrived. But now that it's happening, it feels bitter-sweet, because I may be free from here, but life still feels very . . . very . . . unclear. What am I going to do next?'

'Darling, we have taught you as much as we can about being paralysed, but there is so much more that you will need to learn, and for that matter, unlearn. This is just the beginning. Whatever happens next, Sophie, just try and remember to look after your body because we only have one, and although you might not think it, given how much your body has changed, it's kept you alive, and you have a lot of living yet to do.' Gary stood and gave me a long hug, knowing how to hold me up so that I could hug him back without losing my balance. 'And please also look after that mum of yours, tell her she is one in a million.'

'Tell her yourself, she'll be in to get me in a couple of days.'

'Oh no, darling girl, I don't like to say goodbyes. I became a nurse for that very reason.'

'You helped me rebuild myself, Gary. I really do love you so much.'

'I know I have, but that's my job, now I'm out of here before I start bawling . . .'

Moments after he left, my phone rang. I had kept it off for so long that I barely recognised the ringtone. I looked down at the screen and nearly lost my balance.

Rory.

Aside from the letter he had sent me, I had heard nothing from him, and so upset by his disappearance and unsettled by my growing need to hear from him, I had decided to try to forget he existed. And it had worked, for the most part, but, I pinched myself, I wasn't in one of my dreams, the phone was ringing and it had his name on it.

'Hello?' I braced myself for his voice. One thing the manual hadn't prepared me for was how to speak to the boy you lusted after so furiously, you fucking paralysed yourself.

'Hey, Sophie.' My breath quickened as he spoke my name.

'How are you? I'm sorry I haven't been able to come to see you yet.' He was breathing into the phone, so close it felt like he was inside me. 'But I'm coming south tomorrow, so ... ' There were a few seconds of silence. I thought back to the first moment we kissed, in the snow. My heart pounded, my cheeks flushed, but the rest of me remained silent.

'Are you coming?' I whispered. *Are you coming?* The same three words that had enticed me to Scotland; the three words held so much significance to me now, I never wanted to hear them again.

'Aye.'

'Do you know where to find me? I'm at the spinal unit in the—'

'Aye, I know.'

'Oh, okay. Great. Good. Cool. I mean, right. Sorry, *when* are you coming?'

'Tomorrow, if that's okay?'

'TOMORROW?' The women in the ward all looked at me. I mouthed *sorry*, and picked my jaw off the floor. 'Okay, great, well, what time then? By yourself or ...?'

'It'll be in the afternoon. Keep your phone on. It's been off for a while, hasn't it?'

'Okay, sure, see you tomorrow then.' *How did he know my phone had been off? Had he tried to call?*

'See ya.'

He hung up the phone and I sat with it still to my ear, frozen solid. I only had a few days left in the hospital, my bags were practically packed and I had just one thing left to do, but dealing with this clusterfuck was not it. I was stunned. The thought of seeing him again made me feel as though every stitch and every wound had just reopened and the delicate, freshly made version of myself was stripped away. As though he had skinned me alive, and underneath was a raw, damaged, scared, weaker version which had been created out of my fire-hot longing for him. The wreck from the car crash, who I had worked so hard to rebuild, was emotionally totalled once again.

I weighed up the outcomes of seeing him.

Rory's opinion about my desirability carried greater weight than Jack's, that much was clear by my reaction, and so if he looked at me with the same longing, then that would surely be evidence that the old version of me was alive, and that, even though I was paralysed and using a wheelchair, I might still be her? But if he *didn't* see me that way, then what? Would I have to mourn her more deeply than I knew how?

As far as I could see it, the only other option I had would be to try *not* to put my entire self-worth in his hands – or more accurately in his eyes – but that just simply didn't seem possible. It was more likely that I'd skip out of the hospital later that week than get control of my desperation for him. To be the strong independent self-assured confident woman that my mum would expect me to be felt impossible in this situation. What else was lust if not irrational and stupid? In fact, come to think of it, what else was *love* than a dangerous addiction to the version of yourself that someone else sees in you, that perhaps you can't see in yourself?

But of all the things I had learnt since the night I last stood beside him, running the goddamn world, I did not have the foggiest idea how I could ever find myself again if he didn't see me. My relationship with Jack had run its course; this one, however, had not. Business was still unfinished.

I also suspected that I would look back on the moment and regret just how much power I had given him. So with self-preservation in mind, I decided not to write about it later in my diary, and hope that over time, I would just forget what happened next.

*

The following day I sat on my bed, my chair deliberately hidden out of sight to minimise the impact of seeing me, with my hair washed and my rings on my fidgeting fingers, waiting for him to arrive.

Then suddenly, there he was. No longer imagined but real as day. He walked towards me, leant in and kissed my cheek, and, wishing he would kiss me out of desire, not consolation, I closed my eyes as his lips crossed over mine to reach the other cheek. But he didn't. He looked around for a chair, and unable to find one, sat on the end of my bed sheepishly, looking anywhere but at me.

The conversation between us was a blur to me. I didn't listen to anything he was saying but kept searching for myself in his eyes; instead all I found was evidence that whatever had existed between us once was long gone. And so too, therefore, was I. *Was it all in my imagination? Had he not felt the same? Was it not him who said 'I love you' as I lay trapped under the car?* This wordless conversation grew louder and louder in my mind, but Rory sat opposite me, unaware and, my heart sank, completely unsuspecting. If he was thinking anything similar, I would have never ever known.

There was no denying it any more.

The girl who had once strutted towards him had gone.

All of her arrogance and prowess had been left behind in the crash, stomped into the mud with Mum's high heels, and in their place was a bare confused soul, unable to walk and not yet sure of what or who she was any more.

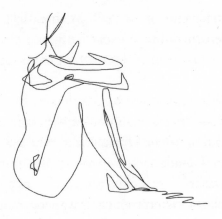

An hour or so later, he leant in to hug me goodbye and as he did, I slipped my hand into the back of his T-shirt, behind his neck, as I used to when we were together. I felt him flinch and saw him glance quickly at me, but then he looked away, and I felt the sliding doors of fate open up. For a split second I wondered what might have happened if we had never met. *What if I had never loved him? What if my attraction to him hadn't been so strong? What if . . .*

I waved him goodbye.

I sat still. Must I dream and always see your face? Suddenly a thought popped into my whirring mind: *Fuck it, it's time.*

I grabbed the bundle I'd stashed in my hospital wardrobe, and before I could hesitate, I reached behind the curtain for my wheelchair, and pushed myself as fast as I could out of the ward, slamming through doors. As I raced down the corridor and past Emma's gym, she waved, but I had no time to stop. Crash, through another set of doors, I pushed over the basketball court and tried to increase my speed. My arms had grown stronger, muscles were forming around my shoulders and neck. My hands had grown rougher. I pushed faster. My wheelchair rushed through the last set of doors, straight into the changing rooms. I didn't even stop to catch my breath. I yanked off my clothes and left them in a pile on the floor.

Ever since I had seen it, I had been thinking about it, and there it was.

I pushed over and clicked on my brakes.

Without hesitating or questioning whether or not I would be able to make it safely, I went for it. My chair slipped from under me but I made it just in time, and transferred neatly across. This was it.

The large plastic waterproof chair was enormous and my rail-thin body rattled as I propelled it. I looked around and it was as I had hoped. There was no one but a lifeguard, who nodded indifferently, no idea what was about to happen.

I took a long deep breath.

I thought: *Here I go. I am going to swim.*

The pool ramp lay in front of me like a runway into the dark blue of the deep end.

I had imagined this moment would take courage, but in the end it didn't. I was ready. I pushed myself forward and watched the water levels rise up my body. The goosebumps on my thighs hinted at the temperature. It didn't unnerve me that I couldn't feel it. I kept on. And then it reached me, the soft licking of the water underneath my breasts. I was in.

Using the arms of the chair to launch myself, I pushed up and away and became separate from the chair.

The water held me as I knew it would.

Without my weight, the pool chair lifted and floated away and then, it was only me. I exhaled and let the air leave my lungs, my breath dropped deep inside my belly, like it had when I'd died. I sunk below the surface and drifted down. It was only me. The tight grip of life tugged me back to the surface but I ignored it, lying below the surface looking up at the ripples as the light broke through. I don't know how long I stayed there but it was a while. Just enough time to work out what I needed to recover myself. Then, as my body begged for breath, I pulled myself up off the bottom and resurfaced.

I took a huge gulp of air and found my balance, using my arms to tread water and keep me afloat. Then I pulled myself into a breaststroke and swam towards the deep end.

The lifeguard watched me and I spun in a circle, just to show someone that I could.

When I got back to my bed that night, my hair dripping wet and a manic grin on my face, I took the Spinal Cord Injury manual and threw it in the bin.

Right, then, I thought, *it's time.*

The last thing I wrote in my diary was: *I think I want to do some extraordinary things, go to some extraordinary places and meet some extraordinary people.*

Watch out world, here I come.

III: THE NEXT

It's Her Funeral, and
I'll Dance if I Want To...

As a mother and a former nurse, in the acute phase of my recovery, Mum's character and skills were put to the ultimate test. Her indomitability had always been apparent, but never more so than when my life hung in the balance. As I had got increasingly weak, she grew stronger and let me siphon off her strength until I was strong enough to begin to mother myself; an act of love that reminded her that no role mattered to her more than being a mum. And it reminded me just how fortunate I was to have *her, Miss Fortune,* as my mum, something I might have never really stopped to consider had my plan to leave the nest and never look back played out.

We recognised that neither of us had expected to have to return to that embryonic, highly dependent mother–daughter dynamic, especially so soon after we'd both assumed the cord between us was about to be cut, so to speak. Still, we had to guarantee my survival, so this dependence continued as I adapted to life outside the spinal unit when I returned home. We didn't need to verbalise how much we wished things were different; that went without saying, at least until the wine came out, that is.

All of my life my parents had presented a united front in

their parenting style. How differently they responded to what had happened to me however, both as parents and as people, was both upsetting and intriguing to me. After my injury, they became two individuals, with distinguishable characteristics, strengths and weaknesses and I began to get to know them.

Unable to understand the language they spoke in the hospital, Dad had been sidelined from the moment the phone call woke them up at four in the morning as Mum stepped into the role of primary caregiver. Dad had cowered behind her, afraid of seeing me paralysed, fearful of his own vulnerability as much as he was of mine so, on the front line of our crisis, Mum and the hospital team took charge while Dad retreated to man the battle station of his office.

But as I recovered and moved into the rehabilitation phase, our relationship in this new life began to define itself. Then, as soon as Dad and I stepped away from the seemingly cold and hostile environment of the spinal unit, he began to defrost, and it was then he saw his opportunity to step up and play to his strengths and be the dad I longed for.

'We all need a bit of *fun*,' he said, hugging me as he cranked up Pink Floyd's 'Comfortably Numb'. 'Let's have a party!'

Now, I know many people would choose *not* to mark the occasion when a person returns home after acquiring a life-altering physical impairment, but for Dad, who is at his happiest on a dance floor, drenched in booze and surrounded by friends, throwing a party seemed the most obvious thing for us to do. And as Dad's love of a party had been hardwired into Mum, Tom and me, how could we disagree, even if I was slightly anxious at the idea of seeing so many people in one place?

As soon as we gave Dad the go-ahead, he took action, calling his closest friends – the ones Tom and I had watched bopping away beside him throughout our childhood – and we all started planning.

'What can we do to help?' had been the soundtrack to my parents' lives since their friends had heard our news, and now, we decided, we would call in their support.

I had booked myself on to a 'multi-activity' weekend with a charity called Back Up, which helps those with spinal cord injury. It occurred to my dad and me that if our friends wanted to help, we could turn the party into a fundraiser for the charity. Altruism – a trait none of us would have ever known we had, nor one we would have had cause to exercise had my injury not happened – came naturally to Dad, and went hand in hand with his hospitable nature, and, I was relieved to see, it put a spring back in his step.

For Mum, the party had a more complex agenda. She wanted everyone to know that what had happened to me, and to her, would not destroy us. Of all the names a person might be called behind their back, 'victim' was the only one Mum really cared about.

Word soon got out about our plans.

My primary school donated a playing field and a marquee, and within no time, a hundred of our nearest and dearest received invitations.

'If we are going to celebrate the worst thing to have ever happened to us,' Dad said, 'we might as well do it in style.' So we decided to make the thing black-tie.

In all the fuss, I didn't find time to think about how I really felt about the party. Seeing Dad so purposeful and focused was a relief, and as the plans took shape, the mood in our home grew more and more upbeat, the music went on and the wine flowed, and so even if I was nervous about seeing so many people or feeling pressured to be cheerful, I didn't entertain those thoughts. I was too busy familiarising myself with old territory and adapting to life outside the hospital. Mum continued to help me when I needed her, but for the most part, my body was in my hands and so my hands were too full for me to think about much else. A week before the party, however, I finally put my finger on what the party meant for me. I felt as though I was being given a chance to go to my own funeral – in a good way. I would see all the people who mattered, all at the same time, all under one roof, and tell them how much they all meant to me. It could act as a proper 'love in', to officially induct these friends into my family, for life. I was being given a second chance at life, and the party would mark my return, and then send me on my way.

So, what to wear? What *do* you wear to your own funeral?

Having lived in a grey tracksuit for over three months, I was completely overwhelmed. I'd never had much of a taste for dresses before, and any that I owned certainly didn't look right on me sitting down: the fabrics bunched up in all the wrong places or got caught up in my wheels when I tried to turn, spin or wheelie. Any I pulled on from my cupboard, I quickly yanked off. They carried too many memories, anyway; there wasn't one that I hadn't once had sex in, and that rubbed me up the wrong way.

Jack was about to leave, and had sent a text message to say that he wouldn't be coming back. Anything that reminded me of our relationship – dresses I had worn with him, underwear he had loved, jewellery he had given me – I had boxed up and packed away at the back of my cupboard, in the hope this act of self-care might help achieve the same with any stray, yearning, unrequited feelings of want for a partner. Of course, the mental clutter was far harder to tidy up than the physical, but I was doing my best. So much of my identity was tangled up in being his girlfriend, being *a* girlfriend, I felt naked without a partner, more naked than I did without a suitable wardrobe.

I asked Mum to help me find a new dress for the party. I decided black, because I was stuck on the funeral theme, and backless, because, well, I wasn't dead after all. I was very much alive. Alive, just not kicking.

Trying to work out what to wear on my feet was also proving tricky: shoes seemed harder than clothes to make fit.

I went through the same selection process as I had the day before my crash, and sat in Mum's closet pulling out her heels, but this time, instead of selecting a pair that could withstand me strutting, skipping, squatting and jumping, they needed to stay both on my paralysed feet and on the footplate of my wheelchair. I pulled off the Ugg boots I had lived in for months and got to work, but either the heels were too tall and my flaccid ankles collapsed, or the soles were too slippery to stay on the wheelchair footplate, or the straps didn't hold the shoes on to my paralysed feet. Like a kick in the face, I realised that the last time I walked may well have been the last time I would be able to wear high heels. But then again, why did it matter? Would I *need* to wear heels when I was sitting down?

'I say you go barefoot, Phie,' Mum said as she planted a kiss on the blonde crown of my head. Decision made.

But a little black dress was never going to do all the work that was necessary for me to feel comfortable that night. When I sat in my wheelchair looking at my reflection in the mirror on the day of the party, my eyes were drawn first to my asymmetric face – my crooked nose with a pink fading scar down the middle, the bulge in one eye socket and the lopsided cheekbones – and then to the lump in my collar bone. As I spun myself around to look at my profile, the twenty centimetre scar stood out in the centre of my back and then, of course, there was the wheelchair: that was impossible to overlook. My body was stronger than I had seen it in months, but nothing could hold in the paralysed stomach or untoned thighs, and my bare feet and toes, perched slightly oddly on the footplate, looked limp. As always, when I looked at them I tried to wiggle them, a habit I so desperately wanted to quit.

I imagined *her* standing where I sat, standing tall in those kitten heels she had selected, and I missed her, I missed her body, the height of her, the physical strength and power of her. I missed her confidence and self-assuredness. I missed that brazen, cocky way of hers. Would she approve of this dress? How would *she* enter a room in a wheelchair?

When I arrived at the party, I found out that it takes me approximately two glasses of champagne, a glass of white wine and two cigarettes till I stop worrying about being in a wheelchair around my friends and family – and a further half-bottle of wine before absolutely no fucks are given. Thankfully, this magical recipe for pseudo confidence kicked in just as it was time for me to step up. I slapped on my best smile and pushed myself clumsily on to the dance floor; Tom lifted me out of my wheelchair and on to a tall chair, and then I poured out my heart, tearfully but merrily thanking everyone in the room for supporting my family and me through our darkest days. My concluding mumbles on how the 'fuck I got to be so fuckin' lucky' were drowned out by a standing ovation, which, I told the crowd with a hiccup, was *ironic*, and then the music came on, and the party got underway.

Dad invited everyone up to dance, and as they rushed in, I was relieved to find the guard that had been up had completely come down. Tom picked me up and spun me around in his arms and it was like the two of us were no different to the two little kids eavesdropping from the stairs, except that here we were nearly adults ourselves. Back in my chair, dizzily, I yanked everyone I could reach down to my eye height to hug, kiss and thank, and when the time eventually came for us to go home, I fell on to the dance floor in a happy heap with Antonia, Sophia and Ellie, screaming Joe Cockers' 'With a Little Help From my Friends', and Boner untangled us; she picked up one of my legs and Sophia retrieved my other leg, and as they lifted my ass off the floor, Boner went one way and Sophia the other, and my legs were spread apart like the splits. We howled with laughter, and all fell over again.

Like a stuck record, I kept repeating it was the 'best night of my life', the *best*, and it truly was, because it was the first night of its kind in this new life, and I was drunk, on white wine and copious lashings of gratitude.

To choose to be celebrating instead of commiserating at such a dark time in your life helps to shine a light into the areas of yourself that might otherwise have been forgotten. It showed me that many parts of me had not been paralysed. The fun-lover who got high on doing the opposite of whatever people expected from her was still in me; she had turned up on the dance floor at some point in the night, and again when I realised that, unable to walk, I could drink anyone under the table! Yes, I may have only rediscovered her at the bottom of a bottle, but give it time and who knew, maybe one day I might recover her completely, even when sober.

My family was putting itself back together, and roles were evolving out of latent qualities in us that may well have lain dormant had we not all been thrown such a curveball.

What my role would be, however, I had yet to figure out.

Kissing a Man in a Wheelchair

'It's a weekend for paralysed people, Mum; why do you *think* I'm packing alcohol?'

The boot of my car was completely rammed. I mentally checked items off my list: sleeping bag, wetsuit, disposable gloves, map, swimming costume, towel, wine. I did some catheter-maths in my head and doubled it, making sure I had more than enough to cover the three days and nights I'd be away, and checked the time. It would be the longest drive I had done by myself and the longest time away. I was driving to the 'multi-activity weekend' hosted by Back Up, in a centre for outdoor activities, four hours away in Devon.

Mum was twitching, checking over what I'd packed, recounting my catheters.

'This paralysed bird is leaving the nest . . .' I laughed, doing my best to put her at ease as I closed the boot. But a flash of worry crossed her face. The trauma had undoubtedly left a mark on her; I saw it every day in the pained look in her eyes and I heard it in the rattling of sleeping pills in her handbag: she and Dad were unable to sleep past four in the morning any more. I knew that they, like me, would carry that moment at the core of them for ever.

We had all passed into a new phase, one which might be

considered the 'aftermath' now the initial drama of the crash had passed. Dad and Mum had returned to work, Tom was back at school, my friends at uni or work; the days resumed, but only with a superficial sheen of normality.

For me, each day was a reinvention of myself and a fortification of my iron will to keep on making progress, physically and mentally, but adjusting to life at home was every bit as testing as the Herculean challenges I had faced in rehabilitation.

Adapting to an inaccessible world was exhausting. The amount of energy required to keep problem solving – working out what to do when there was no accessible toilet or someone was parked in a disabled bay – meant that at times, my frustrations leaked out of me. I still carried the same inherent belief that being independent and self-reliant defined me, and that anything less was a sign of weakness, but life as a wheelchair user required me to be interdependent around my people, and while it didn't come naturally to me, I had to work out how to get around it without it leaving me feeling depleted. The more gracious and well-meaning everyone was, the more guilty and uncomfortable I became, especially if I lost my sense of humour. There are only so many times that the phrase 'shit happens' can be used to make light of a bowel accident.

In hospital my goals had revolved around my physicality; now that I was home, they shifted into working out how to relate to those around me, but there was nothing to guide me. I was on my own in traversing the tricky inaccessible path back to normality, whatever that was.

I quickly learnt to keep quiet when any of my friends or family complained over the smallest inconvenience – the pain of bursting for a wee or shoes being too tight – as I felt enough of a burden and was certain that if there was one way to lose friends and alienate myself, it would be to alert those close to me to how small their inconveniences were compared to being paralysed and in a wheelchair.

It was, I felt, incongruent with basic logic; you wouldn't tell someone their hunger didn't count because there was someone else hungrier. Or someone might be happier than you, so your happiness wasn't significant. Everyone's suffering is relative. Bursting for a wee *is* inconvenient. I just didn't want to hear about it, as much as I was sure people around me didn't want to hear about my problems.

I kept my struggles to myself. If I wet myself, I laughed; if I fell, I swallowed my tears and asked for help with some semblance of nonchalance; if someone spoke about sex, I averted my eyes. I was terrified I might be left behind otherwise.

And around ambulant people an unwelcome question kept being triggered, and it was starting to do my head in: *Why me? Why me and why not any of them?* I wondered bitterly, as I watched them go about their lives.

This unhelpful sabotaging little thought couldn't help but nag at me and as the months passed, it became clear that what I needed was to be around others in my situation. And that was how I had come to choose the activity weekend.

The cover of the charity brochure was what had sold it to me. It featured a woman, around my age, her muscular arm wrapped around a scruffy-looking blond man, both of them in sunglasses and in wheelchairs, laughing with their heads tilted back, covered in mud. I knew a thing or two about fake smiles by that point, and I trusted that these two were for real. I wanted to know them and I wanted to be them. I wasn't looking for new friends exactly, but I was looking to find an authentic smile.

According to the Back Up brochure, every four hours spinal cord injury paralyses somebody in the UK. When I graduated from rehabilitation, I had become one of an estimated fifty thousand others like me but, back at home navigating a non-disabled world, this felt like a completely unrelatable statistic. I was the first disabled person most of my people had ever met, and I worried about the consequences of that.

But, leaving the nest again came with conditions and while Mum was the first to encourage me to go for the adventure weekend, her angst about me driving to Devon made the days in the run-up to the weekend unbearable. Managing her emotions had meant I didn't have time to sit with my own, but I knew that as soon as I was in that driver's seat, I'd be okay. Quite apart from the potential thrills awaiting me at my destination, driving was the only place I felt like myself.

Transferring clumsily into the driver's seat, I wound my car seat back to create as much space as possible for me to pass my wheelchair through. I compressed the pin in the centre of the closest wheel, and then pulled off one wheel, passing that over and on to the back seat, and then I reached over and disconnected the other wheel. The frame of my chair clattered noisily on to the ground. After I passed the wheel into the back seat I then leant out of the car, holding on to the steering wheel for balance, and lifted the frame off the floor and attempted to pass it over my lap and on to the passenger seat. Mum could see I was struggling a bit so she came over to help. 'I have to do this by myself, Mum,' I told her. 'When I stop to get petrol, I'll have to manage by myself, won't I? And when I get out at the other end of the journey. So, thank you, but I'd rather get some practice in.' She held back, testily. Mum hated standing around doing nothing, watching me struggle. The process was clunky and slow, and I managed to hit myself over the head a few times, but after a few swear words and a heave, the frame of the chair made it to the passenger seat and I secured it with the seat belt. I then positioned myself squarely in the driver's seat and did my own seat belt, pausing, but only for a split second, as the belt crossed the centre of my body at the level of my spinal injury. 'I'll text you when I get there. Try not to worry, Mum ... What's the worst that can happen, eh?'

'Sophie,' she said, 'don't make jokes like that.' And she stood on the road waving at me until I was out of sight. I made sure to honk the horn for a definitive goodbye.

With the window wound back up, in the warm cocoon of my car, I cranked up the volume – The Prodigy's 'Breathe' – and hit the road, sighing with relief, singing with all the noise I could muster. With no one around to witness my joy, it felt odd. I turned the music up louder and joined the motorway. *If a paraplegic laughs by herself and no one is around to hear her, does she even make a sound?* I thought. Away from people's perceptions, I felt unsure.

As my little car slipped into the traffic, with my wheelchair tucked neatly (and discreetly) on the passenger seat, I realised that for the first time in a long time, I felt content. The tension and pressure I'd been feeling for so long began to lift.

A few hours later I arrived. I flung the car door open and began the process of disembarking. 'It took me a while to get the process down too,' I heard someone say. 'Do you want some tips?' Looking around, a man, balancing on his back wheels and rolling smoothly towards me, looked so much like Jack I nearly dropped my wheel. Of all the activities I had planned for, getting the hots for a wheelchair user was not one of them. On the way, I'd discovered, as a paralysed driver, drive-thru McDonald's were my new favourite convenience, but suddenly conscious I might be covered in ketchup, I rapidly wiped my face. 'Yes, please,' I said. 'I'd *love* some help! I mean, I've got the hang of it, but I'm so slow and I'd like to get out of the car before the weekend is over ...'

'I'm Tony,' he said, rolling around beside me, 'one of the instructors for the weekend.' He leant on the open car door, crossed his arms and looked at me cheekily. 'You *are* new to this, aren't you?'

'I'm Sophie, and yes, I am.' I tried to attach the wheel to the frame of the chair, but it wasn't clicking in. 'It's so hard trying to keep my balance and lean out to do this ...'

'What level are you?'

'Um, I'm a thoracic, er, level five or six ...' No one had asked me that before.

'I'm a T-12 complete,' he said matter-of-factly, taking over the assembling of my chair. 'I've been injured for about two years, been volunteering with Back Up for about six months. I did this same course myself, so I know what you're feeling right now.'

I doubt it, I thought naughtily.

'It's gonna be a fun weekend, and the weather is set to be perfect. Hope you brought some sunscreen, and a swimming costume.'

A few minutes later I was out of the car, my bag on my lap, pushing alongside Tony to the terrace, where about twenty wheelchair users and a handful of volunteers were gathered in the sun drinking beer. Tony introduced me to them all and I split off to find a space to join the group. After a quick scan, I spotted two of the youngest and rolled over to say hello.

'Hi,' said the woman with a wide beaming smile, 'I'm Maya, T-12 complete, a year ago; I fell off a roof.'

'And I'm Leo,' said the slender, scruffy young man next to her, 'a T-5 incomplete. I had transverse myelitis last summer.' He passed me a beer.

'Sophie, T-6 complete, car accident, five months ago.' Introducing myself with these facts was oddly satisfying. So much said in so few words. And in those brief sentences, already it was as though we'd known each other for years.

The weekend was everything I'd hoped it would be. We asked each other *everything* and anything. Nothing was off limits. When we went kayaking, we talked about sex. When we went abseiling, we talked about catheters. When we hand-cycled for miles, we talked about our families. We talked about what had happened to us, what we used to be like, what we were missing, who we were missing, what we felt, how we felt.

We were all newly injured and finding our way in the world, so we took wild guesses about what we would do next, but mostly we discussed the newness of our bodies and tried to make sense of what we were learning every single day, and let one another dwell on the past and how different our lives were and could have been.

Around other paralysed people my metrics for life soon shifted. If I wet myself I didn't laugh; if I fell, I didn't feel so embarrassed or berate myself, and if we talked about sex, I leant in, curiously. I felt as though I had found a missing piece of the most complicated puzzle imaginable. Being with people who had suffered similar trauma and acquired a similar impairment unified us in a way that went beyond average friendship. So much was communicated without having to find the words for what we had experienced, we could relate to one another's emotions so honestly. And certainly, none of us felt pity for one another.

The common ground we shared was a welcome respite for me.

But in the same way everyone's suffering is relative, so too were our experiences of our individual traumas – we would each have our unique challenges going forward and we debated the advantages and disadvantages hypothetically as the weekend went on.

The three of us were teenagers, so predictably one subject dominated: we talked constantly about dating. We tried to predict what a lover, and possibly even a partner, might look like for one another. Maya thought that women didn't mind being carried or pushed when it came down to it so she and I would have it easier; but men might be too shallow to date women who used wheelchairs, argued Leo, plus men who used wheelchairs were less physically threatening, and that might put him at an advantage. We didn't know. We just enjoyed the guessing. The chats were hopeful, dreamy, and as the weekend progressed, increasingly horny. I found myself watching Tony from the sanctity of my dark sunglasses.

When it was time to go home, I noticed that, no matter how close Leo, Maya and I had become over the weekend, none of us stressed an urgent need to hang out again soon. We didn't want to be around other wheelchair users moving forward; we all had lives that we wanted to return to, regardless of how exhausting it was being paralysed in a walking world, and each of us wanted integration into society, or at the very least, integration into our own individual worlds to start with. I wondered if, after a while, being around other paraplegics would be too intense: a reminder of how different we were to everyone else.

I returned home happier, transferring out of my car effortlessly, smiling at Mum as I told her all about the activities of the weekend, knowing I was ready to move forward in my life, and that if I ever felt alone around my non-disabled friends again, there were friends with spinal injuries I could turn to who would get it.

The best activity, however, I kept to myself: getting to share a kiss with Tony the night before I left, and for the first time, letting myself believe a romantic life – maybe even a sex life – might one day be possible again.

What it feels like to be paralysed

If you are able, place a hand palm down on a flat surface.
Fold your thumb and all of your fingers into your palm, but leave the ring finger extended.

Try to lift your ring finger.

Snowmobiling

Before my car crash, I had never stopped to consider what it was that *really* frightened me. Getting caught doing something stupid scared me but so did fanny farting, so you can see the wide range of my childish concerns. Like many young people, I was fairly fearless, but looking back on it, I hadn't ever experienced *real* fear, nor, therefore, had I tested my ability to override it.

Integrating back into society was far scarier than I assumed it would be. I hated the way people stared at me or didn't see me and the intrusive questions they asked – 'can you still have sex?' – or their ignorant comments –'I would kill myself if I were you' – and day by day, I could feel myself preferring to stay at home and in the protective custody of my friends and family.

Physically, I felt threatened as well. My lack of balance made me wobbly so my eyes never left the ground, scanning for anything and everything that might trip me up, and my double incontinence was intimidating. The thought of not being able to get to a loo in time riddled me with anxiety. I had assumed over time I would find my body less intimidating but the opposite was happening, the more time I spent in my paralysed body, the more it scared me.

All this nervousness could have easily become my greatest

inhibitor, if it were not for one thing. I didn't want to waste the chance I had been given for another life. I wanted to make a life worth living, so I knew I had to learn to overcome my fears. And quickly.

Late one evening, a month after the Back Up course, the phone rang. My parents and I looked to one another, panic-stricken, then all checked the time. Eleven thirty was *definitely* too late for a call on the landline. We were all thinking the same thing: *Tom?*

Dad shook himself out of his panic and jumped up to get it before it rang out.

'Hello? Do you know what time— Oh my God, it's BILL! Bill, how are you?'

Mum and I sighed with relief and settled back on to the sofa. Bill was an old friend of my parents.

'How *great* to hear from you. We are doing GREAT, thank you! Don't worry about the time, what time is it in Canada anyway? The afternoon? Of course! No, no, don't worry, we were all awake,' Dad shouted. 'Yes, yes, Sophie is great, thanks, Bill. Do you want to talk – what? What did you say?' Dad's face lit up. 'OF COURSE, we would *love* to come and see you. When? To visit the Great Lakes?' He looked over to me excitedly and gestured for a reaction. I looked at him blankly. 'Bill, that is so kind of you. No, Sophie has never been to Canada before. No, she has never been on a ski-doo before. Is that even possible? Oh right, thanks for checking. Well, let me talk to her and come back to you. Thanks for calling. Send our love to the family; Carol sends her love too. Okay, speak soon! Bye, Bill!'

They both waited for my reaction.

Of all of the appetites that I was learning to suppress at that time, my wanderlust was proving one of the hardest to ignore. But the various barriers I was facing on a daily basis in my short time out of hospital had already made a deep impact on me, and travelling, or anything that required me to wander outside of my comfort zone, was unnerving. In my mind, the drive to Devon to be with other paraplegics hadn't truly counted because it was a trip designed for people with spinal injury. Flying to Canada to get on a snowmobile did count.

'Let's call Gary and Emma in the morning to see what they think,' Mum said, seeing my mind racing, but when we spoke to Emma the next day, she only confirmed my fears. 'For the record,' she said, her voice straining with care, 'I think it's too soon for you to be travelling so far, Soph. Most people in your situation would still be in hospital. We only let you go home because your mum was a nurse, and you were extraordinarily quick to adapt but . . . ' I could hear the disbelief in her voice. 'Getting on a flight to the other side of the world and going *snowmobiling*, for crying out loud!' Hearing it from Emma made me laugh. It was ridiculous. What was I thinking? 'And flying isn't exactly straightforward.' She then proceeded to tell me how not straightforward it was – the great big barriers of the wheelchair, the relevance of its dimensions and weight, the extra extra time needed to arrive before your flight. 'When you go through security,' she said, 'sometimes you might find your wheelchair causes a bit of a scene, and you'll have to explain that you're not able to stand and walk. They *should* pat you down and check your chair, but be warned, be *patient*, Soph, no swearing, as some airports might try to get you to *stand up*. Then, when it's time for you to board the flight, you'll arrive at the side of the plane in your chair, and you'll be transferred over to an aisle chair, a small chair that will fit down the aisles of the aeroplane because wheelchairs are too wide. They then take your wheelchair away from you, tag it, and put it into the hold with the luggage—'

'But what if I need to go to the loo?' I said.

'This is where flying becomes problematic.' As usual, Emma

wasn't sugar-coating anything. 'Getting to the loo will be impossible for you on your own. You will need to call for the aisle chair, and someone will have to push you. I'm warning you, it's not very dignified.'

'Shall I just put an indwelling catheter in, then? I won't have to worry about anything—'

'Oh no, you will have to worry about *a lot*. An indwelling catheter may prevent you from having to go to the loo and catheterise, but you have to consider your chances of getting a urine infection. In addition to not getting to the loo, you need to think about pressure relief. When you're sitting on an aeroplane seat for so long, you might get a pressure sore, so you will want to take your cushion from your wheelchair and put it on your seat, and make sure you lift every few hours to relieve the pressure. You are also at an increased risk of deep vein thrombosis, so we will need to inject you with an anticoagulant before you board the flight. Your mum can do that for you; get her to speak to Gary.'

'I'll need an *injection*?'

'Yes, to thin the blood, to make sure that you don't get a blood clot from sitting still for so long. Flying is a risky business, and most people in your situation tend to find it very intimidating.'

If Emma was trying to scare me, it was working. But the more I could feel her warning me not to, the more I wanted to. It all sounded doable, just difficult. I was going to have to plan for the worst and hope for the best.

'Er, Em,' I asked, 'what about riding on a snowmobile? Anything I need to think about? Our friend Bill told Dad they're hand-controlled, so I shouldn't have any problem riding one. But it will be near freezing and travelling outside—'

'Sorry to be the bringer of doom,' said Emma, 'but it's not just the cold that you'll have to worry about, Soph. Because you don't know where your weight is, where your *body* is, if you were to lose your balance or slip whilst riding along, there is a very high chance you could fall off, break a leg, heaven forbid. Also, the heat from the machine's engine could burn your legs; the snow could give you chilblains . . . ' She trailed off, having disheartened herself, let alone me, but in the spaces between her words, I had made up my mind.

'Got ya, Em,' I said. 'Lots to think about. Thank you. Look, I know you're worried, but if I am *physically* able to do these things, I can't let my *fear* stop me. Then I'll be even more paralysed than I already am.'

The trip out was every bit as intimidating as Emma had said. Losing my independence, relying on a flight attendant, using a permanent catheter bag, restricting what I ate and drank on such a long flight out of fear of not reaching the bathroom in time, getting an injection, risking my chair being lost or broken, my body being manhandled, my dignity practically stripped from me. It *was* scary, but when I touched down in Canada and found myself still in one piece, my wheelchair also intact despite being stored in the hold with all the bags, I decided it was worth it.

A few days later however, my fear had returned. Sitting astride an enormous snowmobile, beside one of Canada's great lakes, I was shivering and trembling so much I could barely touch the start button.

'Whatever you do, Soph doll,' Bill, a bear of a man, roared at me as he shot off on to the lake on his machine, snow kicking up behind him, 'don't stop, or you might *sink*.'

Dad straddled his snowmobile and revved his engine to follow Bill but waited to make sure I was ready. I checked my legs, checked the throttle. Checked my legs again. They were wrapped in about five layers of clothing and my feet were wedged as tightly as possible into the footwell. I felt for my bum on the seat and checked it was square. I touched the heat of the engine and gave a little prayer that it wouldn't burn my thighs when we got going and it warmed up. I checked my legs again. I pulled down my goggles and gave Dad a terrified smile. This was different to driving; I was exposed to the elements, my feet could fall at any moment, I could become unbalanced. Nor was it like swimming. I was at home in the water. I had never done this before.

The list of reasons why not to drive forward toppled out but there was no time for me to pay attention to the voice in my head.

'Let's go, Dad!'

Dad's machine spun out behind Bill's and into his tracks on to the lake. I pressed the start button, twisted the throttle and jerked forward. The powerful caterpillar tread of the machine beneath me jumped into action, and before I had time to look back to Mum to say goodbye, I was off.

With my eyes fixed on my dad's blue ski jacket, I didn't even check my speed but hugged his snowmobile as closely as possible. He kept turning around to check on me and soon, as the lake opened up, so did our pace. The snow below blurred as we sped up, the green of the pine trees smudged, and all sound filtered down into one deep and rumbling growl of the engines. I'm not even sure how far we had travelled before my senses came back to me, and I got the chance to think. By the time I braved a peek at the speedometer, we were racing at 60 mph, and the shore, with Mum's tiny silhouette, was long gone. We kept going. The speed increased. A bump on the ground made the snowmobile jerk, and my weight shifted dangerously to one side. I couldn't be sure, but I imagined my body twisted out of position because I felt a pull in one direction. I could hear Emma's warning voice in my head but, I reminded myself, she wasn't there; it was just me and the machine. *Just don't stop, just don't stop.* Unable to correct my position without taking my hands off the handlebars, I just kept going. The lake opened up, and the three of us, small buzzing dots in miles and miles of white snow, sped on towards the other shoreline. I didn't know how far it was to the other side. I just kept watching my dad's back. There was no time to think and no time to feel. For the first time since my crash, my mind was still. I was not thinking about the past or worrying about the future. My body and what it could or could not do was forgotten. I was back in the world again. The fresh cold air rushed into my clothes. I twisted the throttle and sped on and gave a tiny little whoop of happiness, my eyes still fixed on my dad.

When we reached the other side, Dad leapt off his machine and ran over to me.

'Mog! My Mog. That was *incredible!*'

His eyes were filled with tears. He hugged me so tight I could feel where my face had been broken. All of the pain and suffering, tireless fighting and adapting, like cobwebs from the past six months, had blown away. My dad and I stayed hugging, laughing and crying, until the feeling came back into our numb hands, and, I suspected, into my somewhat numbed heart.

I had never experienced a rush like it.

Not that long ago, I was so weak that I'd almost died, perhaps I did die at one point. In the near-death experience I came close to *leaving.*

But sitting in the snow on the purring machine, I felt more alive, more present, than ever before, and I paused, looked around me at the grandeur of the snowy peaks and frozen lakes in which I sat, and gave a little thanks to the universe.

Perhaps she isn't such a cunt after all, I thought.

'Again! Dad, we have to go *again!*' I wanted another hit. I *needed* another hit. I'd felt what it was like on the other side of fear, and there was no going back.

Returning home a week later, I was refreshed and revived, like I had shed a skin, and ready for more, wondering just how far I could go next, if I got out of my own way. Experiencing the great outdoors so fresh out of the gate gave me hope. *Where else in the world would I be able to go?*

I wondered what other vehicles existed that could transform my ability to access the world, to take my body where my wheelchair couldn't? From that moment the search began.

The amount of advance preparation for the trip made me worry about how much spontaneity my life might have moving forward, but if the results were to be this rewarding, it was worth being diligent. All the risk assessments could lead towards more risk taking, and it might mean I could start testing my physical limits, and that excited me, as it always had. This time, though, it was more complex than the straightforward adrenalin seeking or risk taking that I'd hurtled towards in the past.

Fear comes in many forms, be it rational or irrational, and as a paraplegic, I was realising that I could find fear in all sorts of unexpected places. But that was what might make my new life so extraordinary. I didn't need to go all the way to Canada and race across a frozen lake to test myself. I could become more courageous through the smallest of acts. All I needed to do was recognise what was frightening me, and if it was holding me back, I should ask myself why I wasn't letting it go.

People often describe themselves as 'being paralysed by fear', and as a paraplegic, I would agree, there is nothing more paralysing than fear – other than paralysis itself, that is. But while one is real, fear, on the other hand, is imagined.

We are born with only two innate fears: the fear of falling and the fear of loud noises. Anything else we are afraid of is learnt, and the most liberating thing about that fact is that almost all our other fears can be unlearnt.

Following My Art

In the 'before', I had visualised what my future life would look like; I'd planned it out, made preparatory sketches in my mind, inspired by the colourful, messy, big lives of people who I perceived to be doing it right. I hoped there would be all sorts of vibrant people in my future, and, most importantly, lots of beautiful places. It would be a life of adventure. The possibilities were endless, the future looked bright, and as far as I was concerned, it was going to be great.

In the 'after', however, the future as I'd imagined it had been washed away. It was lost. I had little idea what was possible.

At nineteen years old, and one year old, my future was essentially a blank canvas.

But as I'd been taught in art, I knew that the best thing to do with a blank canvas was to cover it with colour. It didn't matter what colour you used, or how badly it was slapped on, the best way to start was to just go for it, because the act of making a move was often all that was needed to get your painting going. It was a way of convincing yourself that of all the possibilities available, you had some control over which one you took. After that, you had to use the only tool you had available to tell you that you were headed in the right direction and that tool was joy. If you were *happy* doing what you were doing, then you were on to something.

It was, they say, as simple as that. Or at least, it *should* be.

Growing up, I had always loved painting, but never once had I considered being an artist. Yet no matter how disgruntled I was as a teenager, I was always content in front of a canvas. I lost track of time there, and somehow, everything just made sense. But from the moment I showed a hint of potential in any other area of my education, I'd been dissuaded, the subject dismissed by my teachers as futile. 'She *could* be a lawyer,' my English teacher at school had told my parents and me. 'So that means she *should* be a lawyer,' they concluded, and I went with it because I had the temperament for an argument. I thought I would get off on dominating in a courtroom. But my heart was never in it.

The team at the hospital hadn't discussed my career options with me – that was beyond their remit – but it was generally assumed I would go into the Paralympics. That appeared to everyone to be the most obvious career choice. But I hadn't wanted to take my love of sports further when I wasn't paralysed, so it seemed odd to me to assume that now I was paralysed, a life in sport would entice me. I was confident that I could still play sports for fun; there was no need to dedicate my life to it.

Anyway, it turns out car crashes make for interesting careers advisers.

When I returned home, painting again became a release for my pent-up fury. Art became my medicine and it was obvious that I paid attention to how much pleasure it gave me. I decided to switch my former aspirations for Law School to Art School, and presented my argument for a change in direction to my parents, who, since my crash, only now cared about my overall happiness. And so I won the debate. And soon after, I enrolled in a local art college to do a foundation course. Stepping outside my comfort zone still unnerved me, but after Canada, I had got a taste for pushing myself, a compulsion towards that which scared me. The college was driving distance from my parents' house – close enough to home to have somewhere to retreat to should I run into any difficulty – so I could leave one foot in the comfort zone, and brave one foot out.

But a week before the course was about to start, I was summoned to the college for a meeting. Confused, Mum and I drove there together and as soon as the meeting started I could tell there was a problem. It was explained to us that out of a list of a dozen classes, there was only one that I would be able to access, and also, that there was no wheelchair accessible toilet on the campus.

Mum and I looked at each other, speechless. We had both assumed that wheelchair access would be compulsory.

This is a mistake you only make *once* as a wheelchair user.

'Are you saying,' said my mum softly, the full might of her in the quietness of her tone, 'that my daughter can't attend your college *because* she uses a wheelchair?'

'No, no, no, *no*, we can't, I mean we *aren't* saying that,' said the head of the college. 'She can, of course, do the course. She just can't access most of the campus—'

'Or go to the loo?' I asked.

'No ... I mean, yes. She can't go to the loo on campus.'

Without saying anything, I popped my brakes off my wheelchair and turned to leave. Mum grabbed her bag. Neither of us had ever encountered discrimination this overtly before. The assumption that I had a right to attend college the same as anyone else now appeared to us as desperately naive. It was so shocking that we just left the room without even saying goodbye. Distraught and heartbroken, and stunned by the level of rage I felt, I didn't speak the whole way home. How was it, I asked myself, that I could go snowmobiling across a frozen lake but I couldn't go to the loo at a local city college? How did that make any sense? I had never needed to know my rights before, let alone the laws that protected my rights, but it occurred to me just how urgently I needed to.

As soon as we got home, Mum and I agreed that we needed to get some legal advice so she picked up the phone to our neighbour, who was a lawyer, to ask him for guidance. Furious for me, he said he might have an idea how to help, and to sit tight, he'd call us back the following morning. The rest of the evening I sat chewing my nails, wondering if life was going to be a fight from here on; perhaps it would have been better to become a lawyer after all.

The next day, our neighbour drove into college on my behalf, and calmly and coolly reminded the college that under the Disability Discrimination Act there were meant to be reasonable adjustments made for people with disabilities, but as he understood I was the first student to attend using a wheelchair and adaptations had never been needed, he was sure they would address matters accordingly. Confronted with their failings, they agreed immediately to relocate classes, install ramps and build a wheelchair-accessible toilet.

There were too many old, 'listed' buildings to adapt everything, however – a loophole that confused me as surely disabled people have been around as long as there have been buildings – so when I arrived, beaming from ear to ear a few weeks later, I had to roll in through a back alley, where a couple of homeless heroin-addicts lived, but I didn't mind. I was about to make a mark on my life. I was about to study the only thing that had ever made me happy, and besides, the couple promised me they would keep the path clean of needles and smashed glass. Nothing, not even shards of glass in my palms, could have brought me down at that point.

But it turns out inclusion takes more than a few ramps.

Some of the physical barriers may have been removed at the college, but most of the attitudinal ones remained. The students on my course may have considered themselves to be some of the most progressive young creatives in the country, but for all their vision, few could see past my wheelchair. They pointed at me, even laughed at me, but worst of all, they ignored me.

I had experienced entering a new group in the past, but as the only one with a disability, the scrutiny and sizing up from my peers was fierce. The self-consciousness and severe uneasiness that comes from assuming that if it came down to it, you would be picked last, was new to me. I wanted so badly to make new friends, but without my old ones around for support, to validate me, to speak for me, I felt insecure and uncharacteristically nervous. I didn't know how to change their perceptions of me.

But, making the move, and a mark on the canvas of my life, was significant. I felt empowered. I had made a choice and it felt like the right one, because if nothing else, I suspected that honing my creative skills at art school would be prudent; if barriers were going to continue to present themselves at every turn, I would need as much creativity, as much imagination, as I could muster to find or create solutions. And what better than an artist's imagination to call on in times of need? As an artist, perhaps I would be equally, if not better, equipped than any lawyer to create change in this new life.

Envisioning a life with a disability, and actualising that vision, would require imagination, creativity, determination and resilience, but I knew that if I were to be successful at creating a disabled life worth living, then that would be the greatest art I could ever make.

Going Beyond My Boundaries

Snowmobiling in Canada had only partly satiated my hunger for adventure. A year on, I was greedy for more. So when Emma rang to tell me that the BBC had contacted the hospital looking for people with disabilities to go on an expedition to Central America and that she had put me forward, I was out the door on the way to the audition in London before I'd even hung up.

'I thought you would be interested,' she said. I could picture her telling the researcher: *If you're looking for an intrepid, yet ever-so-slightly unhinged paraplegic, I know just your gal.*

Mum dropped me off at the audition. By now we'd come to an understanding that her opinion on my life choices was welcome and respected, but unless I asked for it, I didn't need to hear it. Having seen me flying across a frozen lake at sixty miles an hour, she appreciated I wasn't going to live within her – or anyone else's – expectations. She knew I wanted to find out what I was capable of and wasn't going to let anything get in my way. She respected my drive to prove people wrong, because that same drive had always existed in her.

It helped enormously, however, that I shot her a reassuring wink before I went inside.

On arrival, I was directed to a conference room, where a table of four young laid-back-looking people sat waiting for me. They smiled as I parked my wheelchair in front of them and took a deep breath.

'Morning,' they chimed and introduced themselves cheerily, by name and title.

'Hello,' I replied. Nerves fluttered in my chest at the thought of stepping into the unknown again, and I was still very self-conscious around new people. 'I'm Sophie.'

'Yes, we've heard a lot about you from your physio, Emma, is it? Well, Sophie, we are looking for a group of people with a range of disabilities and ages, from different backgrounds to take part in an expedition across Central America. Nicaragua, to be exact. The trip will take around a month and will be televised in four hour-long episodes at prime time on the BBC, in a series called *Beyond Boundaries*. We're selecting a group of eleven men and women with a range of sensory and physical impairments to join our expedition leader, a former army officer, as well as an expedition doctor, multiple fixers and some armed guards to lean on for protection. It will be an intense expedition, across rainforests, deserts, rivers and a volcano, in searing heat. Two hundred and twenty miles, from the Mosquito Coast on the Atlantic all the way to the Pacific coast in just one month—'

'To say this will be a "game changer" is an understatement,' one of them jumped in. 'Nothing like this has ever been seen on TV before!'

'So, what do you think?'

'Well,' I said, my heart hammering out a yes, 'I love to travel.'

'Great, can you tell us more? '

'Okay, so, I did a few expeditions when I was growing up in Scotland, camping and walking through the Highlands. I loved that so much. Erm, last year I went to India—'

' . . . but have you travelled *since* your injury?'

'Yes! Yes, I have!' Desperate to impress, I was delighted to be able to tell them I had. 'Yes! I went to Canada and I went on a snowmobile – by myself – across a frozen lake! It was very special . . . I felt very . . . free. Oh, and I know how to get on an aeroplane now.'

'Right.' They looked a little concerned. 'Is that it?'

'Well, I was only injured a year ago . . .'

'Right . . .'

This riled me. I wanted to impress them, but if they didn't know just how hard it was to travel or to fly as a wheelchair user and as a paraplegic then I had no idea how to.

'Sophie, this is going to be a *challenge*. Perhaps you aren't ready—'

Before I could stop myself, a cocky look slapped across my face and I erupted.

'I know I haven't been injured long,' I said, everything to play for, 'but I don't think you understand just how capable I am. I don't even *think* of myself as *disabled*. Emma has helped me to be as independent as possible. I can drive myself around, go to college, and I go out with my friends *and* I went on a multi-activity course and . . . erm . . . Look, what I've just been through since my crash was hell and I reckon I can cope with anything after that. You have to give me this chance to show you what I can do. Please.'

At the time, I was certain that my little rant was what convinced the production company I was more than capable of undertaking the trek in a wheelchair as a freshly injured paraplegic. In hindsight I think it's more probable that this outburst struck what I now know to be called 'TV Gold'. Young, confident and totally unaware, clueless yet courageous Sophie would make for some compelling viewing, they must have thought when I rolled out of the audition, because not long after, the call came to say that I had landed a place on the team.

The timing could not have been better. I had finished my

foundation course and had secured a place at university to study a degree in Fine Art in London later that year, and I realised, in addition to my travel bug being fed, there were several more doors opening. The costs and fear of travelling as a wheelchair user were prohibitive, but under the wing of the TV production, I wouldn't have to worry about either. My hand was going to be held when it came to the logistics of planning and accommodation and, best of all, the costs would be covered. I was living on disability benefits and the bank of Mum and Dad at that point and TV, I thought, rubbing my palms together, could be the ultimate ticket to travel. Even more enticing, I could see that there was potential here; I had so much to show people about this new life I was living. I wanted to share with viewers all the things I had got wrong about people like me, and all the ways in which I was surpassing my own and others' expectations.

The cherry on the cake was that I was going to be trying something new, going beyond my own boundaries. I had never been to a jungle, or to Central America; I had never been on TV or travelled such an unbeaten trail.

It could be the trip of a lifetime.

I didn't ask for anyone's opinion on what I was about to do, not even my family's. Thankfully the production company had helped convince them that I would be safe and in good hands, which saved me the job of exhaustively reassuring them I would be fine, and my friends I mostly kept in the dark, excited for them to watch when the show aired on TV. In the months running up to our departure I didn't think about anything other than stepping out into the unknown once more, and this time, taking the world with me.

But in all my excitement, and planning for the best, I completely forgot to prepare myself for the worst.

*

The team of travellers were loaded on to a plane to take us out into the jungle on the east coast of Nicaragua. I rolled on and took my place, leaving my bags to be loaded underneath. Unlike a normal aeroplane I was permitted to travel in my wheelchair, which was a four-wheeled device designed specifically for the trip, and as I parked up at the back of the hangar, my eyes bulged, all around me were wheelchair parts, prosthetic legs, camera kits and backpacks and I realised I was sitting among the most diverse and unique group of people I had ever met. I had to stop myself from staring, but like a kid in a sweet shop I couldn't help myself.

There was Toby, who had been electrocuted a few years earlier and lost his hand, he told me, as he polished his hook. Carl, who had lost his leg in a boat propeller. Then there was Lorraine, whose cackle could be heard even over the sound of the engines; a motorcyclist had hit her when she was younger and she had lost her leg, but by far my favourite two were Amar, a travel business owner who had a visual impairment – who told me he would always be able to tell where I was by my perfume and my clinking rings – and Ade, a wheelchair basketball player, who had come up with the idea for the show in the first place. He had the most contagious smile and positive attitude. He had contracted polio at a young age and used a wheelchair naturally, as though he had been born into one.

At first, the expedition became a fact-finding mission for me. Unlike the newly injured friends I had made through Back Up, the team had all lived with their impairments for years, some had been born with theirs, others had acquired theirs, and unlike college, where I had been the odd one out, in this group we were all outliers. I couldn't believe my luck. I had found what I'd been looking for in the hospital: a team of people like me, a team to lean on and learn from.

Questions poured out of me and they willingly shared their

stories with me, lives lived to the fullest extent, filled with all sorts of achievements. They each touched on the complexity of living with an impairment, but at the same time, their lives seemed not dissimilar to non-disabled lives. Some worked, some were married, some parents; some were lovely, and some weren't so lovely. They were a group of human beings, but just not your average human beings, and for me, without doubt, these individuals were about as inspirational as they could get.

None of us wanted to be limited by others' perceptions of our disabilities. The same motivation to disprove the misconceptions about what it meant to be disabled was what had driven each of us to apply and I presumed would inspire each of us to keep going.

Entering the jungle on the first night, I couldn't believe the sounds, smells, the heat, the cameras. It was all fascinating. That night, I lay on my camp bed, listening to the howler monkeys in the canopy of the trees above and it was hard to imagine the body I was in was once so lifeless and close to death. I breathed in the dank, succulent air of the rainforest and exhaled with one long happy sigh.

We had a two-hundred-mile mission ahead of us and a month to get from the east to the west coast of the country, so a certain number of miles would need to be covered per day and we had only each other to depend upon, along with a handful of local guides and one expedition leader, a former army officer, Ken. The show wasn't a competition but an expedition, and yet for me, the former was implicit. I was not going to quit, no matter what.

Each morning we set off before sunrise, and I whistled and sang as we cut our way through the undergrowth of the jungle, stopping only to catheterise in a bottle or check my skin for any injuries. The team dug out a hole in the ground and popped a portable commode chair over the top of it for me to use every morning, and within no time, I found a rhythm.

Our individual roles soon became clear, with those of us who could walk helping to push those of us who couldn't, and the group trudged through the jungle merrily as one, following Ken and the guides and gaining ground slowly but surely. If we were to have any hope of crossing the country and arriving at the Pacific Ocean in just four weeks' time, we had to work as a team.

I soaked up as much information from them as I could and scribbled it down in my diary.

The tone Ade used when asking others to push him when he just couldn't manage himself, or the way Amar humbly conceded when he was wrongly accused of not pulling his weight. Lorraine's theories about accepting her amputation around men was so helpful, as was hearing about the way Jane never thought of herself as disabled in her successful role as a doctor back home. I loved how Toby laughed so honestly about his stubbornness as an amputee, he reminded me of myself.

Spending time with these resilient people felt like an achievement. They were the bravest, toughest types of people out there; and it wasn't merely that they were there to prove themselves, it was the fact that their attitudes were so positive in the face of such adversity. I hadn't met people like this before. They embodied so many of the values that I had grown up believing mattered most: they liked to get dirty, to push themselves, to help other people, to challenge themselves, to be part of a team.

But as the days went by, the team began to tire.

We were taking a route very few tourists, let alone ones with any mobility or sensory impairments, would choose. It took us through dense jungle lined with mud and deep ravines, topped with a canopy in which huge snakes could be seen coiled in the sunshine above. Spiders the size of a palm lined my mosquito net at night, and the swollen bites on our arms, proof that we were trekking through the 'Mosquito Coast', grew infected. Trees tangled with vines lined our route and all around were flowers and plants of such vibrancy I wished I had time to stop and draw them. But there was no stopping. We were flanked by armed guards at all times, who kept reminding us that it was best not to delay – rumours of drug traffickers spread like Chinese whispers.

Amar donated his strong body to help me, and in turn I gave him my eyes, guiding him as he pushed me along. At night I would help him orientate himself in the camp, mapping out routes so he could navigate from his tent to the camp toilets independently; in the day, he helped me to wheel over the many otherwise insurmountable obstacles.

But as we progressed through the country, the terrain became harder and harder for us all to manage.

Four-wheeled jungle chairs had been specially designed for Ade and me to use instead of our normal wheelchairs but mine was too heavy for me to push by myself. As I became more dependent on others, the label *burden* clung to me like sweat. This was not what I wanted. I wanted to show how brave and independent I was, not how incapable and dependent I was.

I tried my hardest to find the right tone in my voice to ask for a push or express gratitude instead of anger when the team voiced their frustrations or exhaustion at having to help me, but my conditioning fought against me. Hearing myself plead for a shove or beg for a pull felt horrendous, compounded further by the fact that all of my struggles were being filmed.

When I heard one of the team refer to himself as my 'slave', I broke down in tears. And as we left the jungle, and reached the dry lands of the countryside, my ability to cope in the heat began to wobble even more. In the weeks before the expedition we had all been tested physiologically, and even been put through some assault courses in the English countryside, but these efforts seemed farcical in the depths of the Nicaraguan jungle.

When stronger and more physically able members of the group were forced to return home due to illness, I realised that in my efforts to prove myself, I had pushed myself far beyond my own boundaries. Far too far.

The team around me could see just how much I wanted to complete the challenge, but my refusal to say the word 'can't' soon started to halt our progress. I decided to stop eating because I couldn't risk diarrhoea. My body started to show signs of fatigue. I fought against it as I'd once fought against fear, in the hope that I could overcome it, but my spasms only increased, a sign that I could be in pain or, worst of all, getting ill.

As we crossed into a tree graveyard, fallen timber as far as the eye could see, my chair crashed down over each hurdle and the metal rods and screws in my spine from the spinal fusion began to ache. In one last attempt to keep up with the team, I suggested the team leader strap me on to him and we ride a horse over the terrain, but after a mile strapped precariously on to a saddle, with my inside thighs red raw and my metalwork crunching painfully, it was clear I was entirely out of my depth and would soon have to admit defeat. I came face-to-face with my paralysis.

I couldn't bear that my body was letting me down in this way.

Soon, my unabashed, unshakeable certainty of success came crumbling down in a tearful display of realisation and hope-lessness. 'I don't belong in this body,' I said, a camera pushed into my face. I laid into my unresponsive legs, pinching them to 'wake up, please wake up'. Tears were sliding down my cheeks. 'I don't want to be paralysed any more,' I said, as the camera kept rolling.

*

Up until that point I had believed that all I needed was a positive attitude and to find a way to override my fears, and then, almost anything would be achievable. *'The only disability in life,'* I'd written in my diary less than a month earlier, *'is a bad attitude.'* But while a person's attitude, fears, or even their impairments might get in the way, when faced with one of the most inaccessible environments on the planet, I learnt the hard way that ultimately it is the world around us that truly disables us. No amount of smiling could have got me to the Pacific Ocean, I was physically incapable of completing the challenge at that time.

And then, three weeks into the expedition, I got amoebic dysentery and a urinary tract infection, fainted, face-planted out of my chair and had to be evacuated to hospital.

But before the team moved on without me, a cameraman poked his head into the car where I sat in a nappy, waiting to be taken to hospital, and he asked me what I had learnt. My young sunburnt face looked at the camera and said, somewhat defiantly, 'The best thing I have learnt is that there are some things that I *cannot* do.'

When I'd left the spinal unit I knew that there was so much I needed to learn about living with a spinal injury, so I had seen this expedition as a way to test myself. I also wanted to show others just how much people like me are capable of. I wanted to use the experience to help me to redefine what it meant to live with a disability, and hoped that by going beyond my own, and others', expectations, I would be able to change people's minds, as well as expand my own.

But how much was I carrying from my former life that was influencing what goals I was setting in this life? And whose expectations was I trying to challenge? In contrast to Canada, where I had reaped the reward of overcoming my fears, the jungle had been *too* much of a test.

With the barriers too high for me to overcome, I had set myself up to fail.

But while I may not have achieved what I'd set out to, the experience had given me an insight that I needed at that time: that I was only as capable as my environment was accessible.

When I returned home, I was able to appreciate just how little my impairment disabled me. I could get around in my wheelchair. I could manage my paralysis. I didn't feel like a burden. I had autonomy and agency over my life again.

I knew the best way to move forward would be to continue to push myself, but to make sure I set more achievable, more realistic, goals.

As a person with limited physical potential, my ambitions and aspirations to go further than my own – or others' – expectations after *Beyond Boundaries* had not been deterred, but when the series aired on the BBC a few months later, and I got a call asking if I had ever considered becoming a television presenter, they were then redirected.

Finding Frida

In contrast to the jungle, starting my fine art degree at university in south-east London a few months later was a walk in the park. The campus was accessible and student halls were adapted, so I rolled in composed and ready to go. I'd noticed that I had been upgraded from being called 'the disabled girl' by strangers, to 'the disabled girl off the telly' and it helped me feel a little more confident. I wanted to tackle making new friends head-on this time; even if they did their best to ignore me, I was determined not to be left behind, not to be picked last.

One Sunday afternoon, I pushed myself over to the local pub to find the group of painters whom I most wanted to be a part of. They hadn't invited me but I hoped that if they saw me in the pub, relaxed and joining in, they might see *me*, and not my wheelchair. But before I could get to them, my first hurdle appeared: the goddamn pub itself. Since becoming a wheelchair user, I really hadn't got on well with pubs. They're often inaccessible and they never have any toilets I can use. But everyone loves a pub, so I've had to put up and shut up. Still, I hated them and they seemed to hate me right back. I pushed awkwardly through the heavy double doors and as if on cue, everyone in the pub put their pints down to stare at me. I then got stuck on a wonky step. They then all put their crisps down to gawp at me. I'd spotted the gang of art students at the back, slumped together on a pub bench in the garden, no doubt all in various degrees of hangover from a party I hadn't been invited to. Trying to get to them, my chair wouldn't fit past the tables. The pub all stood and tutted and moved to make room. *Mind your backs*, they shouted at one another. The gang noticed the disturbance. The whole pub was still watching me. 'Fucking *pubs*,' I mumbled to myself. Eventually, I made it to the table and the pub settled down and got back to their pints. 'Hi. Heya,' I said. But no one cared enough to reply. A couple of them were sufficiently alert to at least look embarrassed. I asked one of them to move up and transferred as smoothly as I could from my wheelchair on to the bench, hoping that out of my chair, they might accept me more easily. Suddenly, my body went into an unexpected violent spasm, shaking the pub bench and waking everybody up. They stared at me. I laughed. The spasms kept coming. One of the gang got up and walked away.

I didn't know what was causing my body to convulse, but I knew something was very wrong. I kept my concerns to myself, smiling as best I could to distract from my disability, hoping everything could be ignored.

I eventually discovered the large wooden splinter from the bench that had punctured the skin on my bum cheek and left it swollen and hard to touch. A university nurse removed it and advised me to put a plaster over the area, but I wasn't sure if this was the best thing to do, especially given the wound was in a pressure area, so I planned to go home as soon as my timetable permitted to get Mum's advice.

Back home, a week later, I started sweating and then began vomiting and I passed out. When mum checked the wound, it turned out an abscess had formed. I was rushed to the hospital and taken into surgery.

When I woke up, I was lying on my front, my face squished into the pillow. I tried to turn around, but a nurse stopped me.

'No, don't,' she said. 'You have to stay on your front. You have a dressing on your behind and we can't let you move.'

Groggily I spun my head around to look for Mum. She was talking to a doctor. When she saw me looking, she came walking towards me, and experienced enough by now to be able to read her like a book, I could tell it wasn't good news.

'Phie,' she said, 'the doctors have removed an abscess about four centimetres wide, and now you have a large hole in your bum cheek, like an ice-cream scoop. They suspect the abscess was caused by an allergic reaction to the plaster that the university nurse gave you, but they aren't sure. The doctor says you are going to have to stay "off it", which means lying on your stomach, relieving all pressure from the area, for . . . some time.'

'You can lie on a bed, or on a sofa,' the doctor had joined us, 'but you can't put any *pressure* on the wound. Pressure on it will stop it from healing, you see.'

'So I can't *sit* . . .' I said, trying to make eye contact with him. 'At all?'

'No.'

'But how will I get around?'

He looked at my wheelchair. 'Well, um. You won't. You have to stay *off it*.'

'But for how long?'

'As I told you. For *some* time.'

And just like that, my life shifted on its axis.

Back in recovery, back at my parents' home, I lay on my front, in bed.

The days rotated around the schedule of the district nurses, who came to the house with the punctuality of prison guards each morning. They would peel off the plaster, tweeze out the ribbon of gauze packed tight into the wound, flush it with sterile water then dry, repack, and finish up with a fresh dressing. This took about twenty minutes, all under the watchful eye of my mum, who perched at the end of my bed slugging a cup of coffee, although the coffee was purely a cover. Just as she had done at the spinal unit, she was there to monitor their every move.

The mood was generally upbeat and hopeful, and I kept busy by reading and watching television. I chatted to my friends every so often, and taught myself to knit, presuming that by the time I had made myself a scarf, I would be out and about, and able to wear it.

But the days soon turned to weeks and I realised that there was a reason the doctor had been so reluctant to give me a time frame. The district nurses wouldn't give me one either. I was just told repeatedly that having a spinal injury compromised the healing time considerably. The wound was taking for ever to heal. The metal rods and screws in my spine were starting to ache from lying on my front all day long. Soon, I lost interest in talking to friends and after nearly a month of lying on my stomach, the pain in my spine was stopping me from enjoying reading or watching television. My ability to stay upbeat and positive around my family started to falter, the strain of it too much for me, and my anger which always bubbled away under the surface, was erupting regularly.

Every time they peeled back the plaster, I pushed the nurses for an update.

How much longer? Are we nearly there yet?

'Patients must be *patient*,' the nurses reminded me, as patiently as they could.

No matter how hard I tried, I couldn't find a comfortable position. Lying on my stomach all day was torturous. Confused by the horizontal arrangement of my insides, all food settled undigested, my belly swelled. Stabbing pains pierced through the rods in my spine as though being nailed to my bed. I wasn't even able to sit up to wash and had to go back to bed baths. My only break from lying prone for twenty-four hours of every day was when I was allowed to sit up to catheterise into a bottle or if I needed to manage my bowels, then I was permitted to transfer on to my chair, roll myself, light-headed, to the bathroom and lift myself on to the toilet, careful not to bang my sore or pull off the dressing. During these reliefs I would lean forward and hug my knees, arch my spine convexly and feel my body sing with release. But only ever for a minute.

One minute sitting 'on it', the nurses warned me, equates to one day lying 'off it'.

So I'd do my business hurriedly and rush back to my bed, returning to my face-down position.

Eventually the nurses stopped knocking each morning. Trying not to wake me up, they would tiptoe into my room, and peel back the duvet, and get to work on my wound dressing, hoping my paralysis would render me oblivious to what they were doing to my lower body. But it didn't. I may not have been able to feel, but I could tell what was happening.

Sleeping brought no relief and I never felt rested. I lay in a half-sleep all day and eventually, with the lack of routine or exercise of any kind, I lost track of time. The days themselves were scrubbed clean, nameless and blank for me to fill.

But what do you do with an empty day when you can't move?

Another month went by.

The wound was healing, but it was so deep the skin needed time to knit together from the bottom up. Unable to predict how long the bed-rest would last, I thought it would be sensible to defer my degree for a year, so I called the university and made plans for the following academic year.

The world continued without me.

I would be back soon, I heard myself assure people over the phone, avoiding asking what they were up to, asking instead for recommendations for TV shows to fill my time or books to help me escape. But my friends didn't have recommendations for me because they didn't need to fill their days like this. Their days were overflowing with possibilities, packed with potential. They were studying; they were earning money. Lives were being led outside their beds, outside their front doors, in the world.

How, I don't know, but I remained patient and tried not to think, but I grew sadder and more uncomfortable by the hour.

Nearly six months later, still on my front, I strained over the side of my bed one morning, trying to hear the conversation taking place in the kitchen below my bedroom. I knew it was a decision maker as the last time the nurse had checked, she'd said the wound looked as good as ready. But there had been an unusual redness around it that had been a cause for concern.

I held my breath, trying to still my heartbeat so I could hear. Silence. I swallowed my breath once more and squeezed my eyes closed to help my ears stretch out further. Mum asked a question. It was brief. Silence again. My heart started pounding louder. My eyes began to fill with water. This wasn't how the conversation was meant to go. Where were the laughter and raised voices, the whoops and cries of joy? The sound of a champagne cork hitting the ceiling? Instead, a deep murmur filled the gap. Suddenly, footsteps joined in with the talking and next, the sounds began to fade away. Ten footsteps to the front door. Slam. The nurse had left. I waited. What I didn't hear was my mum skipping up the stairs. What I did hear was a dull thud back into the kitchen. Then sobs.

When she came up, she stood with puffy eyes at the doorway. She did her best to rip the plaster off painlessly, outlining the facts like a newsreader. 'The wound hasn't healed correctly, Phie,' she said, 'so it has to be reopened. You'll have to start again.'

'For how long?' I asked. But her pause made me shut off.

Six months turned into a year.

I turned twenty-one.

In some sort of feeble rite of passage, I spent my twenty-first birthday lying on my stomach.

A party was allowed but, I was warned, it would cost me: one night sitting on the wound could set me back a week. I took my chances. Friends from my old life and some from my new life came and I sat with them around a table, listening to their stories. But all I could think about was the wound I was sitting on. We all drank whisky and laughed, and I tried harder not to think about the wound I was sitting on, but how do you ignore the gaping hole that exists both on your body and between you and your friends?

When everyone left, I returned to my bed.

And still the wound persisted.

We experimented with alternative medicines, healing diets and different dressings to try to hurry the healing but the only way to hurry the process was to stay off it and keep doing more of the same. The doctors just kept telling me to wait. They kept reminding me that the healing process was slower for people who were paralysed.

My spine started to show the signs of scoliosis.

I had been lying on my stomach for over four hundred days and still there was no end in sight.

The pain of being left behind mixed in with all the other pains: the deep reds of anger, the poisonous greens of envy, the cold blues of loneliness, the burnt orange of unsatisfied lust; all swirled together into an unrecognisable feeling that seeped out of my four bedroom walls and into the rest of the house, and Mum was covered in it.

When the bed-rest started, she had stopped working and sacrificed her time for me, but to cope with the strain of being my carer, she had fully reverted back into her nursing ways: smoking, drinking and focusing all her energy on fixing things. She fussed, worried, obsessed, and took control of me so entirely we became one person, just as we had done after the crash. In a way this brought us even closer – without her I would have felt far more alone – but the burden of caring for me seemed to be as heavy as if she were physically carrying me within her and it made me want to get away from her. I hated what I was doing to her. I saw how her hair went unwashed in her plait, her clothes went unchanged; I heard her cry, slumped on the floor at the bottom of my bed. She seemed to be close to breaking point.

Mum always used to tell me that having children would ruin your life, and watching her suffering confirmed that she was right. No matter how many times she insisted she wouldn't have life any other way or that I was the best thing that had ever happened to her, I just didn't believe her any more. How could I? Her life, like mine, was in ruins, and all because of *me*.

The worry of not knowing how much more I had left to endure distilled down into a passive, tired indifference in us both. Any thought about what could be next in life was put on hold and our emotions numbed with distractions as banal as possible. We watched films, we watched TV series, we read books. And because of her, I never quite reached rock bottom. Mum wouldn't let me, she held me suspended as though she had me in a harness. I just dangled around waiting, waiting, but never falling, because she had the ropes ready to heave me back up. But really, the weight of me was too much for one person to carry.

Every day, Dad would go to work – a word that became so offensive to Mum she spoke it venomously, as though it could cut you with its selfishness – and every evening he would come home smiling and sweet, yet pointless and ineffective to the cause; unless he could nurse my wound better, he really served no purpose to her. And it struck me just how hard it must be to be a partner to women like Mum at times; to love a woman who says she doesn't *need* anyone when sometimes, like anyone, she does. As a child I used to see her as entirely self-sufficient in so many ways, she had her own back, but at this time of crisis it made me wonder if a woman can be self-reliant *and* interdependent at the same time?

'It's all right for dads,' Mum said to me one morning after he had left the house, 'they don't feel it like mums do. If you get cut, my girl, I bleed. You know? Men don't bleed.'

I didn't agree entirely; I knew my suffering made my dad bleed too, and even more unbearable for him was knowing that, unlike Mum, mentally, he couldn't carry me at that time either.

My brother stayed away.

Alick, who had practically become part of my family since the crash, came to visit when he could but his life was keeping him busy.

The blocks of our family were crumbling.

The first year turned into a second year.

Seven hundred days of being on my stomach.

My unused wheelchair, which was gathering dust in the corner of my bedroom, taunted me – like an escape route I couldn't take, as it was too dangerous and, if attempted, would extend my sentence. The sight of it broke my heart. It reminded me that not only could I not walk any more, I couldn't even sit.

I longed for company, but the energy once reserved for friends had to be repurposed for self-preservation. Besides, friends didn't seem to get what was happening. They just kept repeating that same advice, reminding me to be patient and that it was only a matter of time until I could have my life back.

Lying there, unable to move, time goaded me like a bored toddler. Because even when it stretches out ahead of you indefinitely and apparently all yours, you won't bloody want all that empty time. Not unless you choose it. Time won't have a value unless you give it one. When someone else forces too much time into your hands you find yourself looking to the walls, you find cracks you never noticed, and the clock – did it always make so much noise? – seemed to take a year to tick.

I tried to sit up, but the wound kept breaking down. Any pressure from my bum bone would open it up further, and then I'd be back on my stomach again. I could have sat in my wheelchair with an open wound because I would not have felt the pain, but the nurses kept advising me to wait for it to fully close, wait for the threat to be fully removed before going back out into the world.

I was as low as I had ever been in my life. The misery of lying so still for so long had consumed me and I didn't smile or laugh much any more. I was in constant pain from the metal in my spine. I didn't want to admit to, or face, the word depression, but I knew I was as close to it as I had ever been.

Then one day, someone unexpectedly came to my rescue.

She arrived in the form of a postcard sent from Sophia in Mexico with a note: *She reminds me of you.*

The postcard showed a black-and-white photograph of a young woman with black hair, a bold monobrow across her fierce-looking face, sitting in a wheelchair in front of a blank canvas. She had a cigarette in her hand, and a ring on every finger. She looked at me in a way that sent shivers down my spine. It was the Patron Saint of the Disabled, Mexican artist Frida Kahlo.

Fascinated, I asked Mum to get me a book on Frida. I wanted to know *everything* I could about her and whoa – her story was uncannily similar to mine. In parts, jaw-droppingly so. Frida, who grew up in Coyoacán in Mexico, was involved in a bus accident when she was eighteen years old, and her spine was damaged; she sustained other injuries, too. Having contracted polio as a child, she had a weakened leg, and the combination of the impairments made her ability to move both painful and difficult. As she got older she had to spend months at a time in bed. It was during those difficult periods that she turned to painting.

I could not believe how powerful her paintings were; Frida's pain felt so visceral to me.

One particular painting called *The Broken Column* seemed lifted from my very own imagination. I stared at it for days. The scribbles I had been making in my sketchbook had been cathartic, but Frida's work was inspiring me to paint again.

One day, I asked Dad to help me move my bed around and position a canvas underneath me so I could copy her work. I painted myself just like Frida in *The Broken Column*: topless, strapped in a corset, with my body torn open to reveal a column, cracked and crumbling. In my skin, I copied the nails she had painted piercing hers, repositioning them in the areas I could still feel.

Every day I painted, lying on my stomach with the canvas half under the bed, but I could only last for about an hour before my arms gave up and I would have to stop and rest for a bit, twist on to my side and let the blood flow back into them or the pins and needles subside, and then start again. I painted in this way, all day long, for weeks.

As I painted myself as Frida, I had conversations with her in my mind and she spoke to me in a way no friend ever had or ever could. I thought about how she poured her pain into her paint for us all to understand just how her life really felt. She didn't want our pity; her suffering wasn't something she wanted us to take from her. She showed us her pain and then she showed us the resilience it had gifted her. Her fragility, she said, was not like that of glass, but of a bomb. A *bomb*. I loved that. Her art was a ribbon wrapped around that bomb. Her story and her art told me that, like so many other disabled or chronically ill people, I was going to have to learn how to suffer the situation I was in and as soon as I learnt how to surrender, then I would get stronger. When your freedom of choice is taken away from you, freedom finds you in other ways and in Frida's case she'd escaped through her art, and the reality that she'd painted was mine too: a woman trapped in her body, a woman alone but with the power to heal herself through her artwork.

As soon as my painting of *The Broken Column* was finished, I leant it against the wall of my bedroom to watch over me. The portrait was life size, my body split open, my breasts uncovered, nails in my skin, but it was the face I loved the most. My broken face looked strong in the painting. I even added the final touch of the scar down my nose.

In Frida's version she is painted as crying, but I didn't paint tears. I looked close to tears, but I am *not* crying. That mattered to me.

I was tired of crying.

As soon as I finished *The Broken Column*, I started a fresh painting, splashing the new white canvas with a wash of blue. The only thing I wanted to paint was the fantasy I had been playing on repeat in my stagnant mind for all that time: I painted myself swimming.

As I painted, I recognised that I had lost myself somewhere along the way, but Frida had left me a map to help me find my way back. Because no matter how strong we may believe ourselves to be, no matter how resilient and determined, in some situations, we have no choice but to surrender that fight, to do our best to let go. No matter how much you might want to, you can't *overcome* your disability like you can *override* your fear. Just like sometimes you can't *win the battle* with cancer or keep *fighting* with chronic fatigue. These nonsensical ideals put the responsibility on the person and ignore the fact that no matter how driven you are to survive, sometimes it will not be enough. Sometimes you are the victim of your circumstances and the only choice you are then left with is how you react to them. That is all you can do. You have no other choice.

I absorbed myself in my paintings, escaping into the paint, into the water that I created and my imagined body floating painlessly under the ripples, and the final months passed by without the monotony and sadness of the first, and then after nearly three long and difficult years, finally, I was free.

Get Naked on TV

A month after I was back up, I received a call. 'The BBC are at it again,' said the voice over the phone. 'They're aiming to break new ground, with an unusual new series.' I put down my paintbrush, and concentrated on what he was saying ... 'It's going to be aimed at educating, inspiring and redefining perceptions of disability. We saw you on *Beyond Boundaries* and we think you'd be brilliant on the show. Real TV Gold. The aim of *this* series, Sophie, is to shake up the fashion industry, which is *renowned* for being elitist and obsessed with perfection, two words no one associates with disability, am I right?!'

'Yes,' I said, trying to get a word in.

'The show is called *Britain's Missing Top Model*. It will be a competition between eight disabled women, and the winner will get a spread in a leading women's magazine and a photoshoot with a top photographer. In a world where people are discriminated against because of how they look, the *fashion* world might just be the last bastion of prejudice, and the BBC want to change that. Would you like to apply?'

This TV guy really had my attention. I hadn't given much thought to the fact that the fashion industry was elitist – that was so obvious it almost went without saying – but thinking about it, perhaps I should start wondering why disabled women weren't represented. What *was* that all about? *Why were there no models with disabilities?*

My cogs were turning.

'What do I need to do?' I asked.

'Just get yourself to London,' he said, 'for the audition.'

The call had come just when I needed it. Art school and bed-rest were over, and aside from considering ways to try to sell my paintings, my life was once again a blank canvas. I had been living with my parents for the past three years, and I was only just starting to work out where I would go next, but with no firm plans in place, it was time to start my life again, again.

A few weeks later, I got a call to say that out of the three hundred and fifty women who'd applied, I had been selected.

'Just don't cut your hair off and fuck it up this time, like you did when you were five,' Mum laughed as she hugged me goodbye. After three long and difficult years together, we were both relieved the chapter was finally closed, and a new and completely different one was opening up. I had never seen my mum so thin, so tired or so despondent. I wanted to find a way to cheer her up, but wasn't sure I had enough in me to pick us both up and dust each other off. 'I'll be fine,' she promised me before I drove away; she waved, as she always does, till I was out of sight.

I was thrust into a penthouse apartment in London with seven other women and countless camera crew, and the contrast to how I had been living was extraordinary. It could not have been more different. I was ready and yet, at the same time, totally unprepared.

The group was an eclectic mix, with women who had been born with their impairments and others who had acquired theirs, some with physical and others with sensory impairments, some with hidden and others with visible disabilities. We were all young and hungry and ready to compete. The aim of the show was to test each of us contestants, to find out what we were capable of as models, and then to crown one winner.

The insecurities I brought with me were one thing, but the other, the unconscious beauty standards that I had been conditioned into following, suddenly became heightened in my awareness as the competition got underway. These standards dictated that wonky, broken, floppy, flaccid, paralysed, seated women like me were *not* considered beautiful (I had checked and the women's magazines confirmed this as fact: there was no one who looked like me in any of them). Furthermore, most of the men in my life had validated my suspicions. I was rarely hit on, flirted with, approached or asked out. The last time I felt beautiful was the last time I walked. The last time I felt seen was the evening of my crash.

But I was open to try to redefine these standards, both for myself and – if the show succeeded – for the fashion and beauty industries.

Over the course of several weeks, four judges put us through our paces in a series of challenges designed to single out which of us would be most able to fill the void the fashion industry didn't even know existed.

The first challenge involved us each stripping down into our underwear and sitting or standing in front of the judges. We presented our bodies without make-up or any other masks to hide behind, and from that moment on, I knew that the competition was going to force me to put all my insecurities behind me. If I wanted to win, I must never let my doubts get the better of me.

Bring it on, I thought.

Sitting in my wheelchair, in my underwear, in a shop window for our second challenge, with passers-by honking their car horns, the high street almost grinding to a halt, it was as close to a protest as I had ever experienced. I was turning my body into a statement, being so visible in my wheelchair, and it felt wonderfully disobedient. It felt defiant, and the part of me that had been so invisible for so many years delighted in being so visible.

Every day that I woke up still in the competition I took as an opportunity to challenge the status quo, so when they put me on a catwalk, I tried to show how a wheelchair could exist in that space, pushing my wheels as gracefully and subtly as possible, pulling my best wheelie at the end of the runway, spinning around as though it was natural and effortless. When they asked us to model in haute couture fashion, I tried to show how a paralysed body could carry the extravagant shapes and gaudy colours. When we were challenged to pose with male models, I did all that I could to look sexy, flopping my legs over the man's thighs and leaning seductively into him.

The photos weren't perfect, but every image taken of me or any of the other competitors added to a portfolio I hoped would shake the fashion industry awake, opening people's eyes to the possibility that disabled women could and should be included in this world.

Every week I made it through, another layer of my self-doubt washed away, and the intensity with which I was analysing myself and being analysed by the judges paradoxically began to help me find confidence.

With each challenge, I let the styling teams dress me in whatever outfit they saw fit, revelling in the pleasure of being styled professionally. Surrounded by so many unique bodies, the perfectly toned whole versions of the average woman began to look comparatively boring to me. I started to appreciate the seated, twisted, stunted, curved, mismatched, wobbly, wonky bodies of us all.

Some of the other girls in the competition were amputees, one had lost her arm in a bus crash, and watching them pose reminded me of the statues of ancient goddesses I had studied in art school. Like the *Venus de Milo*, they were so beautiful.

As the weeks passed a new impetus came into play and I found myself really wanting the series to make real and lasting change to the industry.

At the time, there had never been such a radical display of women like us in the media, and as the competition came to an end the conversation around representation intensified. Everyone involved could see that the programme was more than just entertainment; when it aired it could have the power to shift the dial.

For me, the visibility politics of disability representation now felt deeply personal. When I had woken up in a paralysed body, I had believed it to be worth *less* than the body I had had before. In adjusting to the changes, I confused function with value and assumed that the former dictated the latter. The less it could do, the less value it held. This sentiment impacted my ability to respect and love my body. My body had caused me so much suffering I stopped seeing it positively. I'd grown apathetic towards my appearance and, compounded by years of isolation, I had become indifferent. My paralysis didn't even allow me to tone it or control two-thirds of it, and clothes didn't fit properly sitting down, most shoes didn't stay on my feet. When I looked at myself I only saw what had changed: my face was misshapen, my belly untoned and soft, my legs flaccid. I resented it for being so close to what I'd had before but so very different. The damage wasn't possible to hide with make-up or clothes, and I had tried to just learn to accept it but hadn't quite got there. Losing all sensation in most of it had left me detached, and losing so much power over my body, I thought I'd lost the power to be myself. I had internalised the perceptions that I had once had about disabled people, and only as I started to change my attitude towards my body, did I realise how damaging that had been. I had compared my body to my former body, and that had to stop.

Being around women who owned and loved their disabled bodies inspired me to love my own. I started to see myself differently. Instead of disliking the changes, I reframed my image. In spite of all I had done to my body, it was still doing its best to keep me alive. My arms, which had taken on the job of my legs, were strong and muscular. My little legs tolerated me knocking them around as I transferred badly, my bladder held in all the alcohol I filled it with, even my stomach did its best to behave. All the insides of me were doing their jobs, and yes, I might have lost control, movement and sensation in nearly two-thirds of my body, but it could have been worse.

Spending time fine-tuning my adjustment to my paralysis, scrutinising myself, finding out what suited me, my confidence grew and I progressed successfully through, week after week, all the way to the final.

When the final challenge came around, I was, at last, able to look at myself naked in the mirror for the first time since the crash and not look for *her*.

For the last photoshoot of the competition, myself and the one remaining contestant, Kelly, were going to be nude. This would be the first time a woman with a disability had ever modelled nude on national television.

The night before the shoot I sat alone with my sketchbook, closed my eyes and imagined how I wanted to be seen, where I wanted my legs to be, my chair to sit and my body to face and, with a sigh of relief, I realised I knew *exactly* what a woman in a wheelchair could look like now.

I was her.

She was me.

The next day, I did not resurrect the girl in the black high heels from her muddy grave and have her walk with me into the photoshoot, I wasn't trying to be Sharon Stone or even the old me. The photograph that was taken of me and my wheelchair, naked and strong, is a photograph of a *paralysed* woman, a disabled woman, running her own goddamn world. In it I see the strength of a woman who has been broken and then put back together better. I see all the women who have learnt to accept themselves, who see themselves for all that they are and put value on every scar they carry.

I didn't win the competition, but it didn't matter. I would not be stopped in my mission to change how disabled women are represented, because once you experience the transformational power of accurate representation, you can never look back. I wanted to feel that way about myself for the rest of my life. Furthermore, I wanted other women like me to feel the same way too.

Six months later, I set up a consulting company and started banging on doors, be they in the fashion or retail space, imploring the industry to implement change. Using the only skills I had in my armoury, I drew up some ideas. I had a product manufactured – a wheelchair for a mannequin, a prop to help display clothing for wheelchair users whilst also making more visible the presence of disability in society – and, a year later, achieved some success with it. My prop was installed in the window display of a major retailer's flagship store in central London and I sat on the high street asking passers-by what they thought, spurred on by their overwhelmingly positive reactions. One woman, whose mother used a wheelchair, told me that she didn't know that my prop was exactly what her mum needed until she saw it. *You don't know what you don't know*, we laughed.

But with every step forward, there were many steps back, and doors were slammed in my face far more than I could handle. It obviously wasn't enough to say that representation would be the *right* thing to do; I knew I had to convince people it was a *smart* thing to do, and I tried to explain that disabled people had spending power in the billions, that we were the largest untapped market in the world, but while I may have finally discovered my value, and found value in the representation of women like me, the struggle to convince anyone else was real.

'We will always be "seen" to support disability, but we won't ever do it in our windows,' one retailer said, mistakenly copying me into an email. 'Please someone, get rid of her.'

My skin had grown thicker but not thick enough to keep taking these types of punches, and after a time, I started retreating, finding refuge in my painting instead, knowing that one day the industry would come around, and that when they did, I would be ready and waiting.

You can't just 'get rid' of people like me.

Learn from My Mistakes

From the second I sat upright after three years of bed-rest, I hadn't sat still.

The drive to keep going forward had consumed me, and, somewhere along the line, I'd persuaded myself that there was no use in looking back. What was in the past belonged there.

But when, one evening, I watched a report on the news, and discovered that thousands of young people across the country were being left with life-changing injuries due to driving, and that the single biggest killer of young people in the UK was road traffic collisions, everything stopped. I sat still. I really sat still.

There was something about the fact that my crash was a statistic that horrified me. The few memories of that night that I'd stored at the back of my mind started replaying, and once they started, I wasn't able to stop them. I kept wondering: was there a girl out there taking her last steps unknowingly, and could I somehow find a way to save her?

The only way to stop thinking about it so obsessively would be to do the exact opposite of what I'd been doing for the last nine years of my life: to turn around, and look back at what had happened. To face the facts head-on. I felt hesitant, reluctant to delve into the past, for fear of opening old wounds, but my curiosity was far too strong to curb, and before I could stop myself, as though compelled down a runway road, I decided to go back and unpack what had happened the night I crashed to see if there were clues there that could prevent others from doing the same.

The BBC, having broken the news story that had so shocked me, were aware how alarming the problem facing young drivers was and were keen to explore what was happening. I asked if they would be interested in me sharing my story and if we could investigate the issues, and in no time, a documentary was quickly commissioned. And so, nearly ten years after my own crash, I set off on a journey to find out what was happening.

It was 2012 and according to the latest findings, every day over two thousand people were being injured on British roads, and so, along with Steph, a documentary filmmaker, I went to uncover why so many of this number were young people, why one in three deaths were those of under twenty-fives. It was Steph's job to set out the parameters of the report, and as he, and the BBC, were based in Manchester it was decided we should embed ourselves with the local road traffic police so that we could witness first-hand what was happening on the roads around the city. My role, as reporter, was to go where the story took us.

For weeks, whenever the call came that there had been a car crash, Steph went along and if those involved were under twenty-five, he would try to document what had happened, hoping that the circumstances would tell us more about what was going on. If the specifics of the crash matched what we needed, then Steph would call me to join him, and I would rush up to Manchester to interview those involved. Every time the call came through, nausea curdled in my stomach, and flashbacks of my own crash started, leaving me jittery and anxious. The wrecks I saw were devastating and the injured bodies haunting, the investigation taking me into darker and scarier – yet uncannily familiar – territory, into the minds of young people who had no idea how their lives could change in a heartbeat or how they might suffer the consequences of their actions for the rest of their lives.

I interviewed victims of collisions – perpetrators, too – as well as parents and siblings and friends, and after a while a common pattern began to emerge. It was rarely to do with faulty cars, drink driving or unsafe roads. Instead, it seemed that the young adults we spoke to had not been prepared for the road and they'd had no idea of the danger they were in behind a wheel.

But the consequences of their actions were beyond harrowing, and it brought up so many painful memories about my own behaviour. I started to question my motives for doing the documentary: was I trying to heal myself or hurt myself? Any pain or regret I had buried from my own crash had started to resurface, and after spending a heartbreaking day with an eighteen-year-old woman who had killed her passenger – her boyfriend – on a country road late at night, a familiar figure began creeping back into my nightmares. The boy with the cigarette was back.

In the nine-plus years since my crash, I had seen Rory a handful of times, but I always knew to physically or, at the very least, emotionally keep my distance. He was the embodiment of all I had lost sexually, and every time I saw him, it damaged me. Around him, like a frenzied caged animal, *she* screamed for his attention. It was not an easy feeling to contain. And even though years had passed, even the sound of his name could still disable me. I had succeeded in burying him in the back of my mind after all this time. But I realised the more he came to the forefront, business between us needed to be finished.

After a few more weeks deliberating, I decided what I needed to do.

Too afraid to call him, I texted Celia and Rory's younger brother, both of whom I had stayed in touch with since the crash, and arranged to meet them at the place where the party had been held. I explained the premise of the documentary and that I intended to speak to them about what had happened that night. The plan then was to drive in a convoy along the route I had taken – retracing my steps, so to speak – to the place where it had happened, and Steph would come along for the journey.

It was time to go back to the place where I used to walk, back to the Highlands of Scotland.

The aeroplane touched down in Inverness, and as it slid to a stop, taking my insides with it, I was gripped with an anxiety that robbed me of my ability to speak. Steph kept watching me through the corner of his eye, but there was no going back. The BBC had arranged an adapted car and I drove away from the airport and towards the meeting point, towards the past, with almost every inch of me wishing I could turn back around.

An hour later I pulled up at the location where the party had been held all those years ago, and I parked in the exact same place I had parked that night. Turning off the car engine, I felt an eerie sense, a nameless unease. *She* was here somewhere, maybe her high-heel footprints were under the car where I sat trembling, as her ghost walked around the car, jeering at me, and I tried my best to ignore her. But this was the place that she haunted; I was on her territory and I was frightened of her. I didn't think she would want to see me as I was. She would pity me, perhaps think she was better than me, wouldn't she? I wasn't sure. I had relegated her to the past for so long, I'd not let her walk all over me like this since the early days of my injury when she was not long dead, and still had a hold of me.

Nervously, I found myself winding down the window and sniffing, wondering if her sweet perfume might still linger in the air. I closed my eyes and listened: *could I hear her laugh if I listened hard enough, or the crunch of gravel under her feet? Could I remember what it was like to walk, feel, dance and run?*

It was heartbreaking thinking about what had happened to her that night, and the more I sat there, the more I wanted to reverse and leave.

As the others arrived, Steph got out of the car and positioned himself and his camera far enough away so as not to intrude.

Arriving in one car together, Celia, Rory and his brother (only three of them as Jack had moved to New Zealand), my passengers, parked up beside me. I had asked Celia to explain to the others that we needed to pretend the camera wasn't there, but the pull of the lens seemed to be distracting all of us. The pleasantries felt staged as I opened my car door and one by one they leant in to kiss and hug me hello.

When it was Rory's turn, he leant in so close, I thought I was going to vomit. I smiled and gagged all at once.

'Thank you all for coming,' I said, and it felt awkward and unnecessary. I needed to get a grip in order to do my job as a presenter, and so that my heart didn't fucking explode. 'Shall I lead the way?'

The three of them nodded and got back into their car. I signalled to Steph that it was time, and he came back and got into the passenger's seat, his camera packed on to his lap.

'Are you okay to do this, Soph?'

'Of course I am,' I lied.

I turned on the car engine, and pulled out, driving the very same route that I had taken. The road parallel to the runway stretched out ahead of me; Steph's camera blinked at me, Celia's car followed me at a distance. From the depths of my memory the night of the crash came rushing forward, and as I turned towards the place where I had lost control of my car, I remembered *exactly* where it happened. Suddenly, the wheel in my hands felt hot to touch, and then my breath got snatched away from me. I slammed on the brakes. The car of passengers behind, who had kept a respectful distance, crept cautiously closer. Ahead of me, there was a deep semi-circular black slash in the tarmac. I couldn't believe it. A mark from the past. As I looked at the road scar, I felt a phantom tingling in my para-lysed legs. I parked on the side of the road and paused, trying to gather myself, but I felt as though I had run over my own grave. Never had I felt more afraid.

I asked Steph to pass me my wheelchair from the back seat.

With Rory and the camera watching me transfer out of the car, I felt clumsy and painfully self-aware, and just wanted the ground, the scar, to open up and to swallow me whole.

It was a hot, close, windless summer day and yet I shivered as I rolled forwards, deciding to smoke a cigarette, for something to do with my fidgeting hands, which might otherwise have tried to reach out for Rory. The magnetic pull of him, I noticed with a pang of nostalgia in my hollow stomach, was still as strong as it once had been.

The four of us gathered at the road scar, and Steph spun around us, capturing the conversation as the others talked me through what they remembered. But as they described the speed, the noise, the smells, the order of what happened, all I kept thinking about was how close we'd been to Rory's house. It was only two hundred metres from where I'd crashed.

In the secondary conversation that I was having with him, I was crying out to know what might have been. Did *she* make it into his arms and into his bed? And after that, was she satisfied, was business finished? *Did she run away into the sunset and never look back?*

Where did I go next?

But she and I kept silent and did not ask any of these questions.

I may have been back at the place where my lives had been divided, but the portal into the past remained closed.

*

Later that evening, the four of us sat around a table and Steph prompted me to ask how everyone felt about the night we crashed.

'Thank you all for being here today, and for doing this,' I said as the host of this bizarre dinner party. I'd tried to prepare myself in the preceding weeks, but not even three shots of whisky could calm my nerves. 'I know we've never spoken together about what happened,' I went on, 'but I'd like to know how the crash impacted you all.' My voice sounded hollow. For so many years, I had concentrated on the fact that no one had been physically hurt in the crash, but now, after spending so many weeks talking to other survivors, I knew that no one ever truly walks away from a car crash, and I needed to hear how exactly they had been damaged.

No one spoke, but then Rory cleared his throat, breaking the tension. I waited for that dulcet Scottish voice that used to make my knees buckle.

'I was angry with you,' he said, looking at me, through me, 'because you endangered our lives.'

Then, before I could react, Celia continued. 'Yeah, there was a lot of anger at you, and upset ... '

My face started to pulsate. I found myself verbally shitting out my response, saying that 'Of course that would be the case, I would have been angry if it had been the other way around', but I didn't mean that. I was only saying it because I had no idea what else to say. My mind was spinning. I'd never realised that they had been *angry* with me. I had interpreted Rory's disappearance after the crash as a lack of compassion, so self-centred I hadn't once stopped to think that he might have been furious with me for putting his life, and the lives of all my passengers, including his younger brother, in danger. It was like a slap across my face. How selfish I had been to frame his absence in the context of my own suffering, completely misinterpreting his motives. I started rambling, the whisky finally kicking in.

'I hate thinking that I could have done lasting damage to any of you,' I stuttered, 'and in many ways I'm glad it was just me that was hurt ... I deserve what happened to me because I was driving like an idiot. I just thought that the rules didn't apply to me, and that I could make my own rules and do my own thing ...'

As the whisky took hold of me, the conversation began to deteriorate, and Steph called it. He said we had got what we needed.

We may have got what we needed for the documentary, I thought, but had I got what I had been after? Seeing Rory again had dredged up so many old feelings. Every time I'd braved eye contact with him, I'd found myself searching for me in him: the old memory of me walking towards him jogged into play again in my mind, and then got stuck on repeat, forcing me to replace the vision with something fresh, something that reminded me how much time had passed.

But, just like the scar still carved into the road, time doesn't heal all wounds.

Some are too deep to mend.

I could feel that.

Yet reframing his actions in the light of what he had just shared with me, I felt myself moving as close to a semblance of closure of that wound as I'd ever been. My passengers needed an apology from me, and for me to take responsibility not solely for my actions, but for the reactions they had each had.

Any personal 'unfinished' business I thought I had with Rory felt irrelevant. There was much more at stake. The fact was, I nearly killed the first person I ever loved.

How could my intentions – to sleep with him – have led to *such* a different outcome? How did it go all so terribly wrong?

*

When I learnt to drive, I was never given a lesson in how dangerous driving could be. I was like a child ignorantly picking up a gun, clueless of the destruction I could cause. Nor had I been made aware just how my mood could affect the way in which I drove. I was taught in near perfect conditions, perhaps once or twice in the rain, but most of the time it was just me and my instructor in his red BMW, on the quiet country lanes around my school. We never drove late at night or tested my reactions at speed; certainly no loud music or excited drunk passengers were permitted in lessons. I was taught the necessary manoeuvres to pass the test. Reverse parking was about as technical as it got for me, otherwise the driving experience was a calm, straightforward one, which only ever felt intensified when I took the road that ran parallel to the runway and I could feel my foot itching to push down on the accelerator.

I was taught to drive in the same way as thousands of other young people.

When our instructors deemed us ready, we were invited to take our tests. Of course, not every young driver passes first time, but as soon as they are deemed licensable, one in every five new drivers crashes within their first year, suggesting that what they'd been taught was perhaps not fit for purpose.

Many of us seemed to be learning how to drive after we got our licences, and for reckless young adults like me, a crash was inevitable, and an injury almost to be expected. The more stories I heard the more it appeared that what happened in my crash was textbook, almost predictable.

When I left Scotland the next day, my whisky hangover curdled with guilt, I felt worse than I had the day I'd arrived. But I was leaving with a new perspective. What mattered most was realising that, in addition to helping protect young drivers from themselves, I wanted to protect other young people from young drivers like me.

Road safety experts had been trying to enforce restrictions on young drivers for years. Suggestions included limiting the number of passengers, enforcing curfews to prevent driving at night or imposing new speed limit restrictions. But, wasn't this too reactive? Would these measures be necessary if we simply educated young drivers proficiently?

On my return to London, shaken and stirred, I decided to look into this further, attending a series of workshops that were focused on finding new and innovative solutions to help young drivers avoid making the same mistakes I'd made. And what I discovered completely changed my mind about what was happening out on the roads.

A company, specialising in character profiling and behavioural training for fleet drivers that helped large companies vet which types of drivers would be the safest and most trustworthy to employ to carry their goods, had developed some software to enable young drivers to better understand what type of driver they might be and, in turn, provide brain-training to protect them. The software, Drive iQ, was a series of simulated driving experiences that enabled young people to 'drive' virtually from the safety of their computers, and test out various scenarios that they would likely find themselves in once they'd got their licence, revealing not only the range of dangers they might encounter but also how they as individuals would approach those dangers.

The software was designed to deliberately mature the young person's frontal cortex, the part of the brain that is specifically responsible for danger analysis and risk awareness, because research showed that this part of the brain doesn't fully develop until we are at least twenty-five years old. Using this program would effectively train the young driver to think and behave like an older more experienced one, and mitigate the risks and, hopefully, avoid the inevitable.

In many ways, learning that my young brain wasn't capable

of protecting me when I was eighteen was hard to accept, and learning that there were ways to mature us to improve our chances of avoiding danger was harder still. Had I only been educated better, I wondered, could I have avoided the inevitable? *Could I have been saved from myself?*

And while I would never know the answer to those questions, armed with this information I felt compelled to try to protect others from ever having to go through what my passengers and I had gone through.

I was convinced that Drive iQ needed to be given to as many young people as possible. I put my painting and fashion campaigning to one side and, leveraging the small platform I'd created through television, I partnered with the software company, and we started a campaign.

For the next year, I dedicated my life to educating young drivers about the dangers they were in and how they could spot the many avoidable mistakes that we make when we first learn to drive. I spoke in schools around the country, sharing my story with thousands of children, imploring them to learn from my mistakes and to use the software.

Every time I rolled on to a school stage and retold my story as a warning to others, children flinching as I showed them photos of the car I'd been driving, crushed and splattered with my blood, part of me felt as though I was punishing myself by reliving the event, and yet another part found healing.

I started to make a conscious effort never to refer to my car crash as 'an accident'. It's a subtle difference to some, but for me, it mattered hugely. My *crash* may have been an accident by definition, in that it was unfortunate and, technically, unintentional, but there were factors in my behaviour and in my learning that contributed to the crash and had I been better prepared, or had more experience, then my 'accident' could well have been avoided.

My presentation was like a public act of expiation, but as much as I wanted others to learn from my mistakes, my incentives weren't entirely altruistic. I was doing the work to atone for my actions.

No matter how many people I hoped to help, a year of relentless campaigning, replaying the past over and over again, became exhausting and depleting. I couldn't continue doing it for ever but I did feel that in raising awareness, I'd also made some sort of penance to myself and to the people in my car whose lives I'd endangered.

The boy with the cigarette may perennially haunt my dreams, but I rest easier in the hope that my campaigning in schools might have saved just one driver or one passenger from living a similar nightmare.

Be Your Own Superhero

The first time I saw the trailer for the television coverage of the Paralympic Games, it was the summer of 2012, a few months after I had finished filming the BBC documentary – aptly named *Licence to Kill* – and it initially caught my attention as I recognised the streets where it was shot as being not too far from my flat. Intrigued, I watched on, as the footage cut to an empty basketball court and a running track, and then, as the lights flickered on above a swimming pool, a silhouette of a swimmer with dwarfism emerged, followed by a group of wheelchair users throwing a basketball to one another. My eyes widened. I quickly turned up the volume. As the music kicked in, the screen lit up, a punchy soundtrack combined with a montage of exposed, sweating, powerful disabled bodies: athletes with prosthetics sprinting, football players in blindfolds on a pitch, wheelchair racers training in the rain, all interspersed with clips of bombs going off, ultrasounds looking wrong, and – my heart skipped a beat – a car crashing.

'Forget what you thought you knew about strength,' the announcer was saying. 'Forget everything you thought you knew about humans. It's time to do battle; meet the Superhumans.' And then it cut to a line-up of a dozen disabled athletes each sporting the Great Britain Paralympic Team kit, staring defiantly, unapologetically, slightly moodily, at the camera. Like an album cover for the most disabled pop band ever.

As soon as it finished, I pulled up the trailer on my computer and replayed it, and then again, and then once more just to check I wasn't imagining things. I couldn't get enough of it. This was near enough the most sensational representation of disabled people I'd ever seen.

Since when has a disabled person ever been called a 'super-human', let alone on television?

In an instant, I regretted not having gone into the Paralympics. I swam most days, in a public pool local to my home, but purely for exercise. Seeing these disabled athletes portrayed as superhumans, by comparison my efforts felt pathetic. But then again, *I don't think I've got what it takes to be a Paralympian,* I thought lazily, rolling myself a cigarette and rubbing last night's mascara out of my eyes, having not yet been to bed.

I played the trailer again.

The grit and determination represented in *Beyond Boundaries* was in there, as was the disruptive sassiness of *Britain's Missing Top Model,* but because this was a trailer for an event on a global scale, it packed a more impressive punch. And with Channel 4 – the progressive broadcaster who'd created the film that I had just watched five times in a row – covering the Paralympics, if this was just their advert to promote the coverage, I thought, then what on earth would the coverage of the Games themselves be like?

Over the following few weeks, every time I watched the trailer, it felt to me like a call to arms for an impending revolution, and this revolution even had its own soundtrack, appropriately rapped by none other than the voice of the downtrodden and marginalised, Public Enemy. Chuck D's voice sounded to me like it was inciting a rebellion.

'Thank you for letting us be ourselves,' he sang.

If the superhumans were coming so unapologetically and proudly, I wondered, could that mean us mere mortal 'disableds' got to be ourselves now too?

In the run-up to the Games, all over the country, enormous posters and billboards showed disabled athletes with the words 'Thanks for the warm-up', a tongue-in-cheek nod to the Olympics. The Paralympics were coming next, and according to Public Enemy's Flavor Flav and Channel 4, they were coming with attitude.

The profile of the Great British para athletes began to rise in the public eye. Every day newspapers ran a different story about how the superhumans came to be – who they were, what inspired them, what motivated them, what their day-to-day lives looked like – and everyone seemed fascinated to discover who the superhumans were.

Social media teemed with content about Paralympians from all over the world, all of whom would soon be descending upon the Olympic Park that had been built in the East End of London, and accordingly, the city prepared for their arrival. Sporting venues were opened having been designed with disabled people in mind, public transport had been audited for access and maps had been made to help signpost the step-free routes, and some of London's existing infrastructure had even been adjusted to meet the needs of thousands of incoming disabled athletes and spectators alike.

At this point, I had been paralysed for nearly ten years and for the first time in my disabled lifetime, I sensed a shift both in people's attitude towards me and in the ways in which I navigated the city where I lived, worked and played.

As the Games approached, wherever I went, the prevailing awkwardness or indifference that had followed my wheelchair and me around for the past decade appeared to have vanished; strangers engaged with me and there was a genuine curiosity, with no implicit pity, which I hadn't encountered, well, ever. And I liked it.

It was like being flirted with, an experience I had also forgotten.

Access had also improved; a tube line with step-free access ran all the way from my home to the Olympic Park, and the staff working on the transport networks around London welcomed me as though they were expecting me. Shop assistants knew where their accessible changing rooms were all of a sudden, and miraculously weren't keeping stock in them, and everywhere I went, where once I would have been met with sideways glances, now I had full eye contact and nods that said, 'Well hello there, friend, glad to have you with us. And by the way, well done us for being so friendly and accepting of you and your wheelchair, which, if you haven't noticed, we have not made reference to.'

There was definitely room for improvement, but it was better than nothing.

I was left spinning after every interaction, and as though I had just left an abusive relationship, I started to notice just how isolating and hard being a wheelchair user had always been.

To start with, everyday slights and put-downs had grown commonplace. I was often considered incompetent by strangers, or worse, not spoken to at all, questions directed to whomever I was with instead. I was routinely accused of being a faker or a benefit scrounger, and it wasn't uncommon for people to push me out of the way on the street, or even forcibly remove me, pushing my wheelchair out of the way without my consent.

As frequently as I was being falsely accused of taking advantage of the benefit system or blue badge parking, I was also routinely called 'inspiring', seemingly for very little, such as having a job, driving a car, buying milk, going to an illegal rave. I was once called that whilst crossing a restaurant to go to the toilet.

I wondered what exactly I inspired all these people to do.

The intention behind this fuck-awful word might have been well meaning, but the impact was damaging. It revealed a toxic unconscious bias, that people like me are incapable, and that anything we do, literally *anything* we do, no matter how insubstantial, exceeded people's expectations. Being called inspirational was as insulting as any put-down I had experienced.

It may have been over eight years since I first encountered the access barriers at art college, but not much had changed in that time. Disabled facilities were still hard to find; old buildings took advantage of loopholes that kept them exempt from the laws designed to protect disabled people; goods and service providers often failed to accommodate our needs, citing a lack of demand, failing to see that if they were to supply, then demand would follow. At times I tried to fight my battles like I once had, but I couldn't fight all of them. I picked the few I could, and yet still, the punches continued to come, from every angle. My wheelchair was not welcome in most walks of life.

Believe me, in the autumn of 2012, it was extremely refreshing to finally feel seen, therefore, and in such a positive light – like stepping into the sunshine after years of being in the shadows, and, never one to miss a party, I decided that if there was to be an inclusion revolution brought on by the Paralympics, I was going to find a way to be a part of it.

I arranged a meeting with the disability lead at Channel 4 and to my delight was told there was a small opening in the presenting team that had been freshly recruited to front the coverage of the Games. Everyone involved had a disability, making this new pool of talent potentially the first official group of disabled presenters and reporters in the world.

The role I landed may have been minor, but to me it felt like the most exciting job I had ever had; and by the way I pushed myself to work across the Olympic Park on the opening day of the Paralympic Games, you would have thought I was the lead anchor, all dressed up, humming 'Everybody Wants to Rule the World' and smiling like a maniac at everyone I passed. 'Good morning!' I shouted to the park. This was exactly what I needed: a welcome break from talking about my car crash and campaigning for road safety. It was time to look ahead, not back, and I truly believed the Paralympic Games could be the event – the catalyst – to influence a change in people's perceptions of us, that they could potentially redefine what it meant to be disabled, even trigger a movement that could liberate us. My hopes were high, my expectations soaring, and the role I had in this potentially pivotal moment in societal change ...?

I was reading the weather.

The forecast? Full sunshine with a high chance of *change*.

The coverage was an unprecedented success, bringing in the largest television audience Channel 4 had ever had, and the Games themselves were a sell-out. Every sporting event was packed with supporters, the stadiums were crammed with cheering fans and outside the microcosm of the Olympic and Paralympic Park itself, it appeared the whole nation had got behind the Games. School children were dressing up as disabled athletes, making prosthetics out of cardboard boxes, and wheelchairs out of old bikes, and even sporting brands and advertisers jumped on board, using disabled athletes in their campaigns.

As the superhumans raced, ran, rode, swam, pushed, threw or lifted their way into the nation's attention, by extension, so too did the rest of the disabled community. I couldn't move for wheelchairs, crutches, guide dogs, walkers and scooters.

I even got a phone call from Adidas informing me that three of my mannequin wheelchairs would be installed in their flagship store in Oxford Street.

It was a truly heady time.

Yet it was, at the same time, unsettling, and as much as I was lapping up this newly cultivated friendly and accessible environment, I couldn't ignore just how different my lived experience had been before. After years and years of being left out in the cold, I was saddened to admit to myself, I had acclimatised, and grown accustomed to being dehumanised. Somewhere along the way, I had become blind to, or at least tolerant of, the many microaggressions or direct discriminations that previously occurred so regularly in my day-to-day life.

The world outside was changing for the better, and I was embracing and revelling in those changes. Maybe it was time to re-evaluate my own world too, to check to see if any disablism was happening on my own doorstep.

What ableism had I internalised?

In order to keep up in an inaccessible world, I had always stayed close to, and kept safe in, the arms of my best friends. Boner, Sophia, Ellie and Alick, along with a large extended network of friends, were still, almost ten years on, my armour. My social life was hectic, the parties and holidays regular, with lots of dancing and lots of laughing, so much so, I'd made my father proud. I could party with the best of them. But thinking about it, I had grown so accustomed to being the odd one out – the ugly duckling – that there must have been consequences.

The first of these was that within my group, no one seemed to acknowledge my disability. This was something I'd always welcomed, and found emboldening. My friends often told me they *forgot* I was disabled, which I took as a compliment. But was it? My disability was part of who I was and if they didn't see it, did they see me in my entirety?

It wasn't their fault, of course. I had created the monster, so to speak, because from the beginning of my disabled journey, I had downplayed my differences, doing whatever it took to pretend my disability didn't exist around my friends. If they saw me as unchanged, that was an accomplishment. But it meant

I never expected access wherever we went; I never complained when I had to depend on them to carry me around. I had even resorted to wearing indwelling catheters to avoid inconveniencing them if there was no disabled toilet for me, and my bladder had started to show signs of wear and tear, with an increasing number of accidents and infections. I had also started to eat less when staying at friends' inaccessible homes, to reduce my need to access a toilet, and I never put my needs ahead of theirs. I knew they would hate it if they knew about this, so I kept my harmful behaviour secret from them; but what about *me*, what did *I* think of my *own* harmful behaviour?

And it wasn't only in my social life where I suffered silently. When I went to work, consulting with retailers or campaigning in schools, I would often downplay any pain I might be experiencing or any physical tiredness I might have, anything to avoid being considered unfit or unproductive.

Anything not to be considered disabled.

And for years this had served me. I was surviving, I was keeping up. Just.

Sure, I had lost friends along the way, those who didn't understand that my supposedly feeble excuses as to why I didn't turn up to festivals in fields or weddings on beaches were because I couldn't admit that I was worried about wetting myself or worse, due to a lack of disabled facilities, or the fact I only wanted to be around friends – mostly men – who I could trust to carry or help me. I had got used to being called 'let-down Soph' and let it go.

The friends I kept close acted as my shield and my buffer, and I was grateful for their help removing the awkward barriers that so often prevented me from being able to make new friends over the years, and again, this had been more of a help than a hindrance. My nearest and dearest had brokered many additional friendships for me, and against all the odds, one of those friendships had even developed into a long-term relationship.

This one, unlike a handful of other failed relationships since my crash, felt significant. It hadn't fizzled out or ended after the novelty of being considered a hero for dating a wheelchair user wore off.

Before we started dating, the man in question had carried me up three flights of stairs at a house party, and as he lifted me out of my wheelchair, I wanted to lean in and kiss him but weighing up the possibility that he might drop me if I did, I asked him his name instead, and how he came to know our mutual friend, Sophia. A few months later, I learnt that after he had plonked me down on Sophia's bed and gone to fetch me a beer, he had interrogated Sophia on what I could or could not do – yes, she can have sex – and she had wing-womaned successfully enough that when the time came for him to pick me up and carry me into bed for the first time, although I wasn't entirely relaxed, at least I didn't have to kill the mood explaining how my paralysis affected me.

Our relationship evolved over time, and it was casual, and easy. He was kind, he made me laugh, we liked the same people and the same music, and he never made me feel like my paralysis was an issue for him. Even when a member of his family expressed their concerns that he might have to be my carer one day, he shrugged it off and kissed me sweetly, and we pretended to ignore what she had said, and for that, and more, I had grown to love him.

With mutual friends getting engaged, it appeared my life would soon follow that path.

Mum and Sara, however, had made no secret of their concerns about my relationship – specifically, my behaviour *in* my relationship. I was 'settling' and 'enabling a relationship' that, as neither hesitated to tell me, had I not been paralysed, I would not have maintained. They flagged 'potential addiction issues' and felt his behaviour was often anti-social, his sense of humour and work ethic 'incompatible' with mine, and, deep down, I knew they were right. For them the most obvious red flag was my unhappiness. I explained to them, *surely*, it was best to take what I was given, even if we weren't entirely compatible. Disabled, paralysed women like me couldn't just get the men, the love or the sex that they wanted, I told them, so I'd better just put up with it. I told them that if they couldn't get on board with my decision, then we would just have to see less of one another.

I argued back against them, more than I did against my situation.

But they were right. I was faking my way through my life, and pretending that meant I had adapted successfully.

My patience for enduring prejudice began to appear to me as obedience, repulsive submissive compliance, and that *really* didn't sit well with me.

To make matters worse, I'd never explained to my partner that sex as I knew it, as we were taught to know it, no longer satisfied me. To avoid embarrassment, pity or, worse, rejection, I simply faked my pleasure like I had with Jack all those years ago, pretending I could feel more than I could, never admitting that lower than my breasts, my body was completely locked away from me, and anyone else, and I had no idea how to find the key to unlock it.

I had entirely forgotten what an orgasm ever felt like.

My memories had long since worn out and I had thought about contacting Jack to help me remember, but he had a girlfriend and that conversation would never have been permitted.

I hadn't yet found the language or the confidence to have my needs met, and for years I just let it go, grateful that some intimacy had returned to my life. It didn't matter that my expectations and standards were lower; I was willing to bend because, apparently, according to me, I had no other choice.

But during the Games, my partner could tell something was different about me. I stopped asking him his opinion on what I was doing, what I was wearing, what I was thinking. I didn't ask him if he had watched me in the brief moments I was on TV or what he thought about the coverage in general or about the shift in tangible perception I was experiencing. As though I was starting a new painting or deciding which book to read next, his opinion was irrelevant.

A moth doesn't need a partner to leave its cocoon.

And then, as quickly as they had come around, the Paralympic Games finished. TV returned to its regular scheduled programming, the country went back to work, the world returned to normal, and as life as we once knew it resumed, disability faded out of the everyday narrative.

The superhumans departed.

When I went to Adidas to see my wheelchair props on display, they too were gone.

It was like our day in the sun, the fling, was over.

It appeared naive of me to have assumed that change could have been so close to happening.

But regardless of what may or may not have happened to our society since the Games, I had seen the possibilities, I had glimpsed a more inclusive reality, and I didn't need any more excuses to stay in what had been a toxic environment. I didn't need to wait for the revolution to be televised. I was going to start my own. Be my own superhuman. And in my own revolution, my own manifesto for change would permit me – encourage me – to be outspoken, to be difficult and, fuck it, to make a scene, and with so much at stake, my pleasure, my happiness, my rights, there was an urgent need to advocate for myself and others in all areas of my life, whether at work, at home or even in my own bed, or else I risked living a half-life, made of half-truths.

Any disguise that I might have fashioned for myself, to help ensure my disability went unnoticed by my partner, friends or family, or even by society as a whole, needed to be removed and replaced. And here was a revolutionary thought: what if the world in which I lived stopped expecting me, and others like me, to keep bending, adjusting, squashing, downplaying or outright ignoring our needs in order to fit the mould, a mould that didn't fit everyone anyway?

Maybe then people like me wouldn't internalise these harmful ideas. Because make no mistake, that was exactly what was happening. Ableism undoubtedly existed in me, and I needed to stop letting it. I didn't have to tolerate the situation; I didn't have to keep assuming I had no other choice.

Which meant that, when my partner proposed, I didn't need courage to say the one word that had so frequently escaped me, the most uncomfortable yet powerful word in a person's vocabulary. I pulled out my invisible superhuman cloak of empowerment and that's right, I said it, I said 'no' (and 'thank you' because I was brave but not rude!). And if, for one moment, I doubted my actions, if, late at night, those doubts turned to regret, I made sure to repeat that mantra of Sara's, the one she wrote in capital letters on her very last message on social media just before she suffered a heart attack and died, a reminder to all who knew her, to 'carpe that fucking diem'. Because life's too short not to be seized unapologetically, and authentically, as exactly who you are, every single day.

I didn't ever get the chance to tell Sara we had split up, but I imagined she would have been proud. 'Bloody right you shouldn't have married him,' I'm sure she would have said.

Then, when the ten-year anniversary of my crash came around, I knew that milestone needed to be memorialised, and so I designed myself a tattoo.

Full of symbology relevant to my life so far, I decided that the tattoo was to be placed over the scar on my spine. Getting it done was the most excruciating experience of my life; in some parts the needle felt as though it was inking directly on to my nerves, but I welcomed the pain.

It was time to put my newly found inner strength to the test.

Preventing the
Death of Disabled Babies

The report written by Human Rights Watch included a photo of a young woman with a rusty thick chain around her ankle; the other end of the chain was wrapped around a tree. Her ankle was bruised and cut. I looked at it again and shivered. There was something compelling about the image, compelling yet repulsive.

'She is *chained* to that tree,' said the director of the disability rights program at Human Rights Watch, Shantha Rau Barriga.

'It's hard to stomach, isn't it? She's been in that spot for three years.'

I looked up. Three years in one place. I knew a bit about that. But this was beyond anything I could have imagined.

Shantha explained that Human Rights Watch had found disabled people across Ghana, chained up in so-called prayer camps – spiritual healing centres where people go to pray or seek respite because of a major life incident (such as a death in the family, job loss, or a cancer diagnosis) and in this case, because of mental health conditions.

Unable to move, they had to bathe, defecate, urinate, eat and sleep – everything – on the spot where they were chained.

'Shackling or chaining for any length of time basically amounts to torture,' she continued. 'But if you're one of the 2.8

million Ghanaians with a psychosocial disability, your human rights are often forfeited, especially in the many institutions across the country established to "heal" people. We documented violations against children with disabilities as well . . . '

I threw the report on to the coffee table between us and looked around the table. Two young television producers had called the meeting to which Shantha and I had been invited. Kate and Holly, both of whom have disabilities themselves, had read the Human Rights Watch report and wanted to investigate. They'd seen me presenting on *Licence to Kill* and, as a reporter with a disability, they wanted to know if I would be interested in going to Ghana on behalf of the BBC. I had travelled as much as possible over the years, although never to West Africa, and despite witnessing and experiencing discrimination in various forms wherever I went, I had never seen or heard of the types of abuse detailed in the report.

I needed something to throw my energy behind and I was grateful to be given a chance to work in television again, to have a platform to use my newly found voice. But this subject matter was harrowing. Sensing my trepidation, Kate explained.

'We want to document what's happening, and then take it to the Ghanaian government, to see if we can support Human Rights Watch in their effort to put an end to this inhumane practice. Your job will be to find contributors who can speak to the reality of living with a disability in Ghana both to create an educational and informative programme and to try to use the documentary to bring about change. The programme is asking if Ghana is the worst place in the world to be disabled.'

I was all for creating change, I thought.

'Fuck it,' I said. 'I'm in.'

'For Christ sake, Sophie,' Mum said. 'You're going where? The worst place in the world to be disabled? Are you actually trying to kill me?'

'We don't know that yet, Mum,' I said, trying to console her. 'We're just there to ask the question. Also, listen, there's a government grant that will help me cover the costs of someone to accompany me, to help me, you know, push me around, carry my chair or bags or even carry me if necessary, and I'm going to see if that someone could be Tom.'

Ever since my injury, the perception I had of my brother's life had always made me hesitant in asking him for help because, basically, I didn't want to disable it. Tom had established a life for himself that looked uncannily similar to the one I had once dreamt of for myself and in the photos he showed me, I saw my old self, and I desperately didn't want what happened to me to interrupt him.

But as the years passed, that impulse to hide my disability from him had grown into one that sought him out. I wanted him to follow me, join me, as he once had as a kid. So when this Ghana job came up and I knew we'd be filming in inaccessible locations, often without access to toilets or accommodation, I thought about asking my brother to come along to help me physically. Perhaps, too, after all these years, I could finally be a sister he could be proud of.

I had often struggled to find the language needed to ask for help, but I was done pretending not to need support, especially at work. Still, when I called Tom, I was so worried he would say that he was too busy, I opened with the fact the role would be paid, positioning the trip as a job for him, as opposed to help for me, so that were he to say no, it wouldn't hurt my feelings. There was no need.

'Soph,' he said, 'I'm honoured that you've asked me. Of course I'll be there for you. It would be my pleasure.'

The Human Rights Watch report had outlined that Ghana had a number of prayer camps where people with disabilities were taken to be healed and, in some cases, subsequently chained. Given my previous experience with the mind instructor Hratch Ogali, I had my issues with healers of any kind, but our investigation and my role required me to put my cynicism aside, as I would be going undercover into the camps, under the guise that I wanted my spinal injury to be fixed. The cover story was that I was there for healing purposes, and filming it, solely for myself.

It was time to learn the subtle art of being subtle.

The crew, Tom and I touched down in Accra and, getting straight to work, the following day, a local fixer took us to one of the first prayer camps on Human Rights Watch's list.

The camp was on the outskirts of the capital, down a long dirt track. On arrival, a man approached us and welcomed me warmly, directing me to a long queue of people with tired faces – many with crutches and a few in wheelchairs – that was snaking its way inside one of several single-storey, mud-lined buildings. I went to join this queue in the hopes that I could meet the owner of the camp – a self-proclaimed prophet – to find out exactly how she helped people. Our real motive, of course, was to find and, if possible, film how they really treated disabled people, including putting them in chains.

As I pushed my way over towards the queue, a terrifying sound stopped me in my tracks. I looked at Tom. He had heard it too. Then a scream, a sharp piercing wail, filled the compound, practically rattling the car windows.

'It's a child,' I said to the camera. 'There is a child somewhere here, and for some reason, it is screaming.'

From inside one of the buildings, a woman stepped out into the sunshine, pulling a little girl, who was limp in the body. Her eyes bulged and yellow and red snot streamed out of her nostrils. She screamed again, delirious and disorientated, and still holding her up, the woman started to cry. As she walked towards me, dragging her child, she pointed at her face. 'It's medicine, to help her,' she told me in-between frightened sobs. The child's legs gave way and her mother sobbed painfully. 'I am trying to help her.'

In the way she looked at her daughter struggling, I recognised an expression I'd seen so many times on my own mother when I was suffering, and instinctively, I took her hand in an effort to comfort her. I looked around for someone who might help her but the man who had greeted me was nowhere to be seen. The queue of waiting people watched on, as curious about me and the camera crew as I was of them. Aside from the piercing shrieks from the girl, however, no one was making a sound. It was eerily quiet. The cameraman, director and Tom all skirted around me, hovering and scanning for evidence of the shackling, trying to look as inconspicuous as possible, but we stuck out like a sore thumb, and I was anxious our presence would invite questions.

The child's screaming set my teeth on edge. I was agitated about what we might find in the camp and worried about being caught in a lie, but at the same time, maybe all those years of scheming and lying as a girl had prepared me for the role; undercover investigating with a secret microphone wired inside my shirt was an audacious and novel kind of troublemaking.

Tom spotted a building at the far end of the compound and signalled for me to go and look. Reluctantly leaving the girl and her mother behind, I pushed myself towards it and peered into the darkness, the camera followed me over my shoulder. As my eyes adjusted to the dark, I gasped. We had found what we were looking for: men and women of all ages were chained up in the dark.

The smell in the room was stomach churning. Some of the men were openly wanking, one man appeared to be covered in faeces, one woman lay covered in what appeared to be vomit.

As an inexperienced reporter, words failed me.

Suddenly a shout, like a warning, alerted the camp to an incoming threat. I froze and looked for a way out, but there was nowhere to hide. We had been caught.

As though she was perfectly used to seeing a team of foreigners in her prayer camp, one with a television camera and one using a wheelchair, a woman dressed in bold colours sauntered past us towards a young woman who sat chained on the floor, and beat her hard across the face. I was stunned. With no obvious concern about us witnessing it, she slapped her again, looking at the camera, and then at me, as she did it. No one else made a sound. The chained woman cried out as she was struck. Her abuser, who I now assumed to be the self-proclaimed prophet, looked at me unapologetically, as though to say, *Don't worry, I am doing this for her own good.* She handed the woman a concoction and made her drink it.

A shiny new-looking Land Cruiser arrived outside the building, and the owner turned from us, walked outside and took the front passenger seat, her driver fastened her seat belt. Finding my voice after being momentarily mute with shock, I followed after her and tried to speak to her through the car window, asking why so many people were chained in her camp, but her driver signalled for me to be quiet and without another word, the two drove off, leaving me and the crew coughing and spluttering in a cloud of dust.

In addition to witnessing the practice of chaining, and in order to find the answer to the question that had brought us to Ghana in the first place, I needed to unpack what life was really like for people with disabilities. The Human Rights Watch report I had read gave me a comprehensive overview of the reality for people with mental health conditions, but to see the bigger picture of how disabled people were treated generally, I needed as much information as I could get.

We travelled the country and I interviewed as many people as were willing to talk to me – families of children with physical disabilities, men with mobility impairments, women with mental health conditions, charities, aid workers and pastors – and the more I investigated the more I began to paint a clearer picture of why the chaining was happening.

The prevailing perception I encountered was that persons with disabilities were considered cursed or demonised. When a person was born with or acquired a disability – physical, sensory or psychosocial – with so little support or resources available in the community, families often had to turn to prayer camps, who used a range of solutions to try to fix the problem. Prayer, fasting and chaining were all common practice. But when these solutions offered in the camps failed or the costs were prohibitive, alternative treatments might be sought. People talked to me of witch doctors and fetish priests, and their part in the story appeared relevant so, after enquiring into where to find one man in particular, who was rumoured 'to send' disabled babies 'back to the gods', I was directed to meet a local healer who worked not far from the capital city.

Instructed to bring two chickens, a bottle of schnapps and some American dollars, I arrived to meet a man with blood-shot eyes, wearing a dirty red smock and a necklace of cowrie shells. He invited me into his home and, after I handed over the necessary payment, began my consultation. But I wasn't there to find out why I was "cursed" – although he told me I unquestionably was. My job was to understand exactly what he did to the disabled babies that were brought to him. I pressed him through our translator as best as I could, but the situation made me frustrated and was not helped by him insisting that his reading of my situation was hard for me to believe; apparently I was disabled because my parents had tried to kill me. Several heated, sweaty moments later however, he finally explained that what was meant by returning disabled children 'back to the gods', was that he left them by the side of a river to drown.

It's not every day you look into the eyes of a man who murders disabled children.

Tired of me and my indignation, he called off the conversation, and left. So I gave a riled piece to the camera, confused and, in all honesty, out of my depth. My disability had been seen by the BBC as justifying my role as presenter, but the more time we spent on the ground, the more I found being a white British middle-class paraplegic woman afforded me little insight into the reality of living at the intersection of poverty, gender, race and disability in Ghana. But I kept reminding myself that, like any reporter, I had a story to find, a job to do.

The investigation continued.

I met more people, they shared their stories, we filmed and then moved on, and day by day I grew more adept at reporting, which basically meant I grew increasingly numb to what I was seeing.

Then, one afternoon, I was driven to a small village and dropped off inside a compound. In order to keep my interview as authentic and revelatory as possible, I was given no further instructions other than to find a disabled man who lived in the compound and ask him to share his story with me, a story that, according to my director, I could relate to – something to do with bed-rest.

In the corner of the compound sat a woman, smoking, scowling at me as I pushed towards her, but as I neared her, she stood up, stubbed out her cigarette on the floor, turned and walked into a small wooden door tucked in the corner of the compound. She opened the door and out of the darkness a body, carried by two men, was dropped into a plastic chair, right in front of me. A festering stench of rotten human flesh filled the space, so revolting it almost masked the sight of the man himself. Emaciated and distorted, his bony limbs dangled limp over the chair, unable to use any strength to hold himself, his neck rolled wildly, along with his wide petrified eyes, adjusting to the outside like a rabbit in headlights. The compound was completely silent, everyone rooted to the ground, mouths open and staring. They looked as though they had just seen a ghost.

This was worse than anything I had imagined. Why he had been suggested as a contributor was beyond me; he looked as though he had no idea what was happening. I introduced myself to the man, but he looked only at the woman, so through the interpreter, I asked her, his gatekeeper, if it would be okay to speak to him on camera, perhaps inside his room. She repeated my question. He blinked a yes. The man was then carried back inside, and I was ushered in behind him, the camera following.

Inside, the smell of the room was worse than that of his body. The man sat, weak, on a blood- and dirt-stained mattress, piles of rubbish around him. Every inch of me wanted to leave, out of revulsion and respect, but if I wanted to be a reporter, I had to stay. I transferred out of my wheelchair and sat on the ground beside him, deeply uncomfortable at the thought of probing him but curious to understand what had happened. Why did the villagers look as though they had never seen him before? Why was he so emaciated? The interview was staggered and broken but gradually we found a rhythm.

Francis told me he was thirty years old. When he was fifteen, he said his body started feeling tired, exhausted, and shortly after, he noticed his muscles began to deteriorate. No longer able to walk much further than a few metres, he depended on a wheelchair. But he wasn't strong enough to push himself in the heavy metal chair he had been given, and his friends declined to help him. No one wanted to be near him, he said. Unable to afford the prayer camps, his mother decided it was for the best for him that he should stay in this room, and he hadn't been able to leave since.

Francis had been hidden away for fifteen years.

As he spoke, the stink of shame that hung in the air of his room grew more and more evident. Of course I recognised it, I had breathed in that air before myself, most disabled people would have caught a whiff of disablism at one time or another, but I had never known it to be so potent.

Had I just been reporting this story as an impartial news reader then the content I was uncovering may have been easier to relay, but as a physically disabled person who had experienced being confined myself, I felt such empathy for this man it was overwhelming. The scene was so unbearable, the room so oppressive, that despite my attempts to be professional, I started to well up. I thanked Francis for sharing his story with me, and asked him how I or we might be able to help him. It wasn't my place to rescue Francis, but I didn't know how to just leave him in that room. He explained his mother had contacted a charity to try to help source a wheelchair, but from the way he spoke, something told me he wasn't telling the truth. Despair doesn't need to be translated. The fixer told me not to worry, that help would be on its way, but I could not know for certain.

It was time for us to leave. I called for my brother to help me get up from the floor and back into my wheelchair, and those three simple movements emphasised the distinction between Francis and my realities. In the weeks we had been in Ghana, my brother had not left my side, he was my legs when I needed him and a shoulder to lean on throughout, and all the ways in which he supported me was never more apparent or more valuable to me than when I saw them juxtaposed with Francis's situation.

I drove away from him, scanning the doors of every house we passed, wondering how many other disabled people were trapped behind closed doors, and I hoped that in recording his story, he testified to the heartbreaking fact that it wasn't only iron chains trapping disabled people; stigma was every bit as disabling and, worryingly, could never be undone with the turn of a key.

There were two more interviews to conduct before we were to return home.

The first was with a team of young people with physical disabilities, who met in a car park once a week to play skate football. One of the team was a teenager with a leg deformity, who lived in one of the slums outside the capital. As we rolled around the city together, he told me that after he had finished school, his disability had got worse, and despite his qualifications, no one would employ him, so he spent his days begging. I asked him if he had ever been to a prayer camp, or to see a witch doctor or fetish priest, and he said he had been to both, but they weren't able to help him. He didn't go into detail. I asked what he thought about the shackling practices that were happening in his country and he told me, with a smile, that while he didn't know why he had been cursed, he trusted that God had his reasons. Disabled people, he said, deserved their fate.

He had validated his reasoning with a religion that I didn't believe in, but his words resonated with me deeply. I too had once used the word 'deserved' to help me make sense of what had happened to me. I had reasoned my own disability in the same way, and assumed my paralysis was a consequence of my actions, a punishment I deserved because I had been so reckless and selfish as a girl.

But that reasoning now felt inaccurate to me. I didn't believe my disability to be a punishment any more than I agreed disabled people deserved to be tortured or killed. If anything, being paralysed had been rewarding to me. What hadn't killed me had made me so much stronger, and my injury had taught me so much, given me a chance to become a better version of myself. I was turning my suffering into meaning; my life had purpose, I just knew it.

But maybe all these conclusions were only possible in the context of my privilege; had I acquired my disability under different circumstances I might have drawn different ones. And would then I adapt my beliefs to help reason my fate accordingly? Of course I would.

It was not for me, or anyone, to determine what people deserve, but I replied to the Ghanaian man as honestly as I could, saying that the only thing I could say with any certainty was that all any of us truly deserve are basic human rights.

On my final day, I got the chance to put our findings to the secretary of the National Council for Persons with Disabilities, but disappointingly, although not unsurprisingly, he was unable to offer any concrete resolutions on the spot. He admitted the country had done nothing to act on Human Rights Watch's report, and that while they were aware of the killings, and the torture in the camps, little, or not enough, had been done to stop them.

And so, disappointed but hopeful, we left Ghana, determined to make a documentary to show proof of what was happening, in the hopes it would hold those in charge to account, if not by the Ghanaian government, then at least by the international community. Only time would tell if it would make any impact.

Like anyone awoken to their privileges, I returned with a greater appreciation for all that I had, but I noticed a confusion when applying my gratitude in day-to-day life. Any advocacy I wanted to do would have to evolve to try to create change in many different areas of life, not just in the spaces where my life existed. But I felt it imperative that I didn't ever tolerate the comparatively less discriminatory barriers that existed in the

UK – the First World problems, so to speak – because while the discriminations I had experienced in my life felt trivial in contrast to what was happening to disabled people in Ghana, at the same time, they were simply a less extreme version. The injustices against disabled people around the world varied greatly, but every step towards inclusion, no matter how small, still mattered. While I couldn't say for certain that Ghana was the worst place in the world to be disabled (although for television purposes I was directed to say I did think it was), neither could I say that the UK was the best place to be disabled.

Sometime later, when I next saw Shantha, she told me that the report, documentary and courageous advocacy from local activists – many of whom had mental health conditions themselves – had built mounting pressure on the Ghana government, which pledged to investigate the camps. The UN expert on torture visited Ghana himself to see the situation and called out the abuses. Funding for mental health in Ghana increased fourfold. Now it was about how that funding would be used, and local groups, together with Human Rights Watch, continued to push for all mental health efforts to have human rights at their core.

But nothing could be done to save Francis; he had died a few months after we met.

The Reason Trap

F resh back from Ghana, I was determined to pursue a career in television, for a plethora of reasons: I loved how challenging the job was; it paid better than any job I had ever had, and living with a disability was expensive – a lightweight wheelchair cost more than my first car – and from the limited experience I had, television had permitted me to go to places, see things and meet people I would never ordinarily have met, and it gave me a platform from which to speak about, and shine a light on to, the disability experience.

The reactions I had encountered as a wheelchair user at this point had ranged from being considered cursed, my handshake refused for fear of catching something evil, to being asked how many medals I had won in the Paralympics. Presuming I was a superhuman was one thing, but when it came to the other stereotypes, it was another thing entirely. Watching TV, reading the news, scrolling through social media as a non-disabled person, these misperceptions could easily be forgiven. Pedestalled or pitied, superhuman or cursed, perceptions seem to be polar opposites and whichever category we are put in, ultimately, these tropes were traps. Neither left space for disabled people to be average human beings. Representation, in my opinion, needed to be more accurate.

I still believed that television, if used correctly, could be a powerful tool in changing, in correcting, perceptions of disability, or at least as powerful a tool as I could get my hands on to attempt to create the change I wanted to see in the world.

But as a person with a visible disability, presenting roles were few and far between. Unless there was a valid reason for my wheelchair being on screen, it was hard for broadcasters to justify my role as a presenter. I was told repeatedly that there weren't roles 'for wheelchairs' on TV, not unless the subject happened to be about disability.

It all smelt like ableism to me, but still, I persisted.

With the 2016 Rio Paralympic Games fast approaching, an unprecedented window of opportunity opened up for disabled talent and when Channel 4 announced they were recruiting for new disabled people to cover the Games, feeling I might be in with a chance of success, I went for it. I wanted to be part of the coverage that had so moved me in 2012, and not just as a weather girl. I wanted to be part of the Paralympic *movement* and, to be honest, I *really* wanted to go to Rio de Janeiro!

The Paralympic Games were not necessarily the best platform on which to attempt to smash those harmful stereotypes that positioned disabled people as 'inspirations', as *superhumans*; after all, the Games were where we deliberately put disabled people on pedestals, the Games are the epitome of the triumph over tragedy trope, they are 'inspiration porn' for the masses, the personification of the stereotype.

But I also knew that the Paralympics were the greatest, the largest platform available to disabled people to change perceptions. They could, if used correctly, impact our society for the better.

After a challenging week-long audition process, I landed a role as one of the lead anchors, and life as I knew it went into overdrive.

Zooming into the studio in the months leading up to the Games, drum and bass pounding in my headphones, a smile plastered on my face, I arrived for training every morning, raring to go. I was loving, *loving*, what I was doing, loving the potential of it, the hope, the thrill, the glamour and the graft. Live television presenting was without doubt as much fun as I could have with my clothes on *or* off.

Being an integral part of the Paralympic coverage was not an opportunity I was going to fuck up. I approached the training, the preparation and the responsibility as if my life depended on it.

Which, in many ways, it did.

When I was asked to pose in my wheelchair for press photos I put my hands on my wheels, like I was always about to move off, active, on to the next great thing, and I smiled as big a smile as possible, showing people that I had worked out how to embody the label 'disabled'. When I was interviewed for magazines or newspapers, I spoke about myself using words like 'fulfilled' and 'purposeful'.

In my personal life, my relationships were improving and I noticed how comfortable I had become when articulating my needs. I had started dating a friend and our relationship was flourishing. I hoped it had the makings of something great. Many of my old friends were now married, Boner included, or had moved away, Sophia included, and we understood that our paths would naturally start to separate so we let them, connected for ever in the shared tattoos we'd each got at the time when our lives were so intertwined it was impossible to imagine a day without each other.

But new people had come into my life and old relationships had fizzled or burnt out, and my need to be surrounded by people who knew the other me had lessened.

I knew now what I wanted to look like as well, I'd ironed out what clothing worked, finding designers that created adaptive clothes. I'd figured out how I wanted my hair, where I wanted more tattoos, which shoes would stay on my feet, how to transfer almost anywhere, which wheelchair fitted me correctly *and* I'd even found, after years of searching, a motorbike that would be capable of carrying me and my wheelchair.

My ducks, as Mum likes to say, were in a row.

Since the time I had been on bed-rest, I had made a conscious effort not to cause Mum any more suffering. I knew how much she worried about me, but I had learnt enough to look after myself, or at least, I had learnt how to ask other people for help when I needed it. This left Mum and me room to concentrate on the positives, to laugh and relax and enjoy one another's company.

The excitement I saw in her in the run-up to the Games made the role feel even more significant; my success was a gift to my mother, and my father, for all I had put them through. Every time Mum sent me a photo of a newspaper clipping or recorded a radio interview, my guilt lifted a little more.

When the Games began, I sat in the hot seat in Rio, and leapt into eleven days of live broadcasting to an audience of millions, and the lights, the camera, the action, all of it, was electrifying.

For my part, as one of the lead anchors, I wanted to use my role to address the fact that while disabled athletes might be equipped with resilience the likes of which most non-disabled people could only imagine, and they might wield their vulnerabilities into weapons of strength to fight the constant unrelenting ableist forces that look to take their liberties from them, at the end of the day, they were still human beings. So when the athletes arrived in the studio for interviews I deliberately leant into conversations that spoke to the ways their lives could be relatable. I knew that the 'superhuman' disabled athletes, like all of us, had weaknesses, had struggles; some lived on benefits, some campaigned for accessible public transport, some didn't even have access to assistive technologies. They lived on a spectrum of suffering, the same as everyone else.

No two Paralympians were the same, there were athletes with no legs, swimmers with no arms, riders who couldn't speak, powerlifters with dwarfism, sprinters who couldn't see, and with over four thousand athletes from 159 countries each one represented a different experience of disability. Some had been born with their impairments, others had acquired theirs in every way possible, wars, car crashes, shootings, medical malpractice, the list went on, and it was in their commonality, in the details that revealed their shared lived experiences, that their real powers were revealed, as far as I was concerned. I didn't mind how fast they could run in a straight line or hurtle down a pool. What I admired was the fact these types of people saw adversity as an opportunity, found strength where others saw weakness, and refused to be knocked down. That was what made them superhuman.

As broadcasters we also orchestrated a debate on the word 'disabled' itself.

Some athletes rejected it, adopting other terminology, coined to liberate those who saw themselves as a person or an athlete with an impairment (person-first language); others preferred identity-first language (a paraplegic woman or blind sprinter); some preferred the term 'crip' or 'differently-abled'; some even preferred to be called 'diffabled' or 'handicapable', as they felt marginalised and mislabelled by the word disabled, and clearly wanted to smash down the barriers of language in a cry of self-reclamation.

I was down for all of it. As long as it was us who decided what we called ourselves, I could see no reason to argue with anyone wanting to define their own label. After all, I too had once seen 'disabled' as a dirty word, evoking such a visceral sense of weakness it felt incongruent with who I saw myself to be. I had thought that being deaf, blind or paralysed were labels so burdensome, I would never be able to carry one, let alone be proud to be one.

That had, however, changed. I had grown comfortable being called disabled. In fact, I was wearing the word like a medal around my neck.

When the Games came to an end, I made a strategic and deliberate decision to try to use the place I had just earned at the table as one of the few female presenters in the world with a visible disability, to go where very few other disabled presenters before me had gone – to transcend disability programming and make content that didn't make any reference to my disability, didn't use it as a means to 'inspire' viewers or elicit pity in people; my wheelchair, my paralysis, my accident, all of what had happened to me, was to be incidental.

As a presenter, I didn't want to have to come with a warning, or to give my back story, or justify my role through any other means than my talent. I needed to prove my worth. It was important to me to have confidence in my ability to present, and not feel as though my place on screen was purely to tick a diversity box. I didn't mind ticking a box, so long as I ticked it whilst doing my job properly.

Clear on a mission, with my agenda packed and priorities straight, I went to work as a presenter and, without doubt, it became the best job I could've ever imagined.

For the next few years, whether I was travelling around the UK, helping couples settle their differences in a daytime television series about property renovation, heading off to the South Pacific to report a current affairs story about rising obesity rates, embedding in a community in northern Australia to report on disproportionately high rates of indigenous children in the justice system, going undercover to expose tricks in the British restaurant trade or exposing the dirty secrets of the tech giant Amazon, wherever the job took me, I pinched myself. And as my profile grew, I started to use it to create the change I wanted to see in the world.

When Shantha called me to tell me that the BBC documentary had in fact made an even greater impact and that the Ghanaian government was making the practice of shackling illegal, well, if I needed any convincing that I was on the right path in life, this was it. It sealed the deal, put the nail in the coffin, confirmed my suspicions that all of my pain and suffering over the years, and all the ongoing difficulties that came with being paralysed, were worth it. Because if I hadn't had my injury, then I wouldn't be where I was, making a difference. If I was ever to find a reason for why I had been paralysed, this work might be it.

I teamed up with charities that mattered to me, from Back Up to Human Rights Watch, as well as organisations like Leonard Cheshire, which help disabled girls access education in developing countries, or Scope, the disability charity in the UK. Travelling the world, I supported as many causes as I could, advocating for those that might otherwise be left behind. I resurrected my efforts with retailers, consulting with some of the largest in the world, such as Target in the US, to implement changes for disabled customers. I supported companies that were innovating in inclusive travel and design industries. I spoke at the United Nations. I hosted Global Disability Summits. I won and judged prestigious awards for disabled people.

I went, my arms stretched out wide, like the figure in the drawing I had once made in hospital, as far as I could.

My paralysis fitted into my life and became the source of my motivation, and in many ways, my disability came to define so much of who I was.

I had it under my control, or so I thought.

But then, one day, while visiting Ellie at her home in Scotland, I transferred into my wheelchair and slipped. I fell, face first, to the floor. My hands rushed to protect my face, one leg got tangled in the frame of the chair, my body twisted and I crashed down.

Shaken and shocked, I pulled myself up but then my heart stopped, there was blood on the floor beneath me. My heart dropped into my stomach.

I reached around to feel under my bum, and felt for the scar of the old wound. My fingers found it and then returned, covered in fresh red blood.

My sore had just reopened.

Drive Forward

N ow, whenever the wound reopens, regardless of how prepared I try to be for its inevitable return, it's like a bomb going off. I might always plan for the worst and hope for the best, but very little can prepare a person for the moment they come face to face with their own vulnerabilities. Confronting your limitations takes courage, overcoming them takes resilience, and at nearly thirty-six years old, setbacks of this nature, no matter how predictable or familiar, require an untold amount of both.

The last time I had been trapped on bed-rest, I was terrified of being left behind by my friends; but now, it was my career that was at stake.

Lying prone all day long, the wear and tear on my shoulders, crunching metalwork in my spine, and stiff joints, was agonising and painfully demotivating. Unable to sit up, I had to let go of all my presenting work, and try as I might to remain confident that when I returned there would still be a job for me, doubt made me restless. I had progressed in my career, but I hadn't reached the lofty goal of any aspiring presenter: presenting a series of my own. As a disabled woman, I didn't know if that equality of opportunity would extend to include someone like me, certainly I hadn't ever seen a female wheelchair user front their own series, and while I had come close, I had yet to convince any broadcaster that I was capable of carrying my own show. To do so, I needed to find the right idea, one that could demonstrate that my disability could be incidental, and yet at the same time represent myself authentically. I had been trying to level up in my career, but I had always sensed there was a glass ceiling, and now the wound had reopened, I was afraid I would miss my chance to find out if I might be capable of breaking it.

If bed-rest was going to be anywhere near as long as last time – and I had no idea how long it might last – would my career wait for me, or would there be another, younger, less impaired person in the place I had worked so hard to create for myself?

Thankfully, Ellie had given me a room in her home for bed-rest. It came without the heavy guilt or responsibility that my old bedroom in my parents' home had had and, having recently separated from her partner, Ellie welcomed me living with her, insisting she loved the company. My friend slotted my care into the daily routine of her hectic household, into the feeding times, nap times and bedtimes she kept for her three children. Children who, since the day her first son Luca was born, thirteen years earlier, Ellie had always said could be my children too.

I have made the decision not to have children of my own so I love the idea that one day I might be to them – and all my god-children – as Sara was to me: a second mum, especially to Ellie's youngest, her daughter, who, to my delight, she named Frida.

It isn't that I am not able to have children – a few years after my injury I found out the hard way that being paralysed wouldn't stop me from being able to get pregnant – I am just not *willing* to be a mum.

What I want instead is what I have always craved: freedom of choice – something my eighteen-year-old disability was, once again, preventing me from having.

And to add insult to injury, when the bed-rest started, my partner left, and with him gone, some familiar insecurities reappeared, reminding me painfully that though many areas of my life had flourished over the years, some had not, and answers I would have hoped to have found by now regrettably, still remained unknown.

Despite the great efforts I have made to adapt to my paralysis, there remains a hole inside of me due to the fact I have yet to discover the key to my body. Unable to feel two-thirds of myself, no matter how hard I have tried, the act of sex has still not been adapted satisfactorily enough to *fully* meet my needs. Pleasure and intimacy take many forms, I know that to be true, but I can't help but ask myself if it is 'better to have loved and lost than never to have loved at all', and when that applies to sex, I would say the answer for me is an undeniable *no*, it is not better to have had it and lost it.

What I've experienced in 'the after' does not compare to 'the before'.

After Sara died, I vowed to make better choices in my relationships, but no matter how hard I tried, many of the same problems recurred. After several failed attempts to find a partner who could see me entirely, including my wheelchair and my paralysis, I have grown despondent and sadly grateful when a man comes into my life, unable to stop myself from falling for them, simply for being with me, even if they don't really see me. Often, when there has been love on my part, it has been unrequited, or, if I have been loved, it was for the wrong reasons.

The relationships have been difficult, toxic, a few have even been abusive.

Searching for validation in another person has been more detrimental to my well-being than any physical challenge I have had to endure, and my drive to be *seen* by others has distracted me from the far more worthy pursuit of simply existing happily as I am.

But when the world insists on reminding you, every time you go out the front door, that you are lesser, you are other, that you aren't of value, that you aren't worthy of belonging, the work and the strength required to ignore those messages can feel insurmountable. Especially when your own body won't let you live as you want to either.

With my latest relationship now over, nowhere to go, no work to distract me, no parties to escape to and not enough art to medicate me, with nowhere to hide from myself, back on bed-rest once again, I couldn't stop myself from wondering what my life would be like had I *not* been paralysed, what it would be like to be *her* again.

I usually *refuse* to indulge in this fantasy. It is as pointless as asking Ellie or Mum what their lives would be like without their children. The question is redundant, the answer is unknowable or, if guessed, a pipe dream, or a nightmare, that can never be actualised.

Letting my mind take me where I can no longer follow, especially when on bed-rest, can be dangerous. Ever since I had tried so hard to walk again, and the miracle had never happened, I really had used every ounce of my strength to try not to think about *her* too often. I had taken control of the wild child in me. Even when I watched people dance or saw a woman straddle a man, and I felt her stir in me, I had taught her how to sit and stay obediently, like one of Mum's working dogs.

Occasionally I dream about her, but now even my dreams have wheelchairs in them. I have the last photographs of her but don't tend to spend time looking at the young me, the *old* me.

But, what if, *what if,* I could be her again? If I could set *her* free, what would *she* do, just for one day? How would she carpe the fucking diem?

Well, this is what I would do, if I were her.

On waking up in this daydream, first things first, I would *have* to wiggle my toes. I would *watch* them wiggle. *Feel* them wiggle.

Then, I would pull my legs up close, hug them, and then jump up, spin around, before pausing, gathering my breath, then I would leap up, making a star shape as I flew and whoop, I would land, *thump,* on to the floor.

Both feet firm and flat on the ground.

I would stand up, tall.

I would command Underworld to play from the closest speaker at full volume. Flexing every muscle in my body, watching the tendons and the ligaments move to my command, as the music gets louder, I would twist my hips, twist and grind and rotate them; my hands, no longer needed to move me, find their way into my hair, tug and flick it as I jump and dance.

I'd skip outside and push my toes into the nearest soil, feeling the grass and cold dirt on my soles, and then roll, still naked, in the mud.

If my body needed to urinate or defecate, I would let it do so in the dirt; my hands would remain free, letting my body do whatever it needed. Luxuriating in that feeling of release.

I would find the nearest body of water and dip my toe in and remember just how indescribable it feels, and then immerse myself in it.

I would yank on a dress, a dress so long and floaty and free it would feel as though it was barely there.

I would sit down, then stand up again, and then sit and stand up again.

I would run my hands all over my body, from my breasts to my toes, and back again.

Closing my eyes, I would put my hands between my legs, and I would feel myself again. I would keep my hands moving there.

Only when my knees had reminded themselves of what it felt like to be buckled, would I be satisfied and move on.

If the day was mine, and I could fill it as I pleased, I would dance with my brother, ride a horse with my mother, ski down a mountain with my father.

I would hug them all, standing up. We would then raise a toast.

I would put on some black high heels for a moment, and then kick them off, gather all of my friends, and we would all rave, barefoot. I would dance and writhe and handstand and kick and stomp and pound the ground till it hurt.

Never once would I sit down.

I would walk into some woods and have someone, with dirty-brown eyes with flecks of green and rough calloused hands, rip off my clothes and touch me, stroke the skin on my shins, pinch the flesh on my thighs, lick the creases of my body, finger at the insides of me, suck at the tip of me and make me melt with their hands on my belly.

Then, I would straddle them and control the speed and the pace and find the pleasure *I* wanted.

Then, I would walk, by myself, and I would get lost, scrape my legs on the bracken, and eat blackberries from the bushes like I did as a girl, and I'd howl at the fucking moon from the top of a tree.

This is what I would do.

If I was her.

I realise, however, as this forbidden fantasy comes to a close, after seizing this dream day, that I have come so far it is safe to look back, because the girl I once was, the eighteen-year-old me, no matter how much freer she may be able to be than me, I believe at the end of that dream-day, she would look at herself in the mirror, at her unbroken, straight, scarless face, at her tall, strong body, and I believe that she would miss *me*, the other me.

This me.

The one who sits in a wheelchair.

I think she would miss this version; I think she would *prefer* this version, no matter how broken this version might be physically, how disabled, because this version is the best of *us*. The disability might have paralysed *some* parts of her life, but without it, the other parts may never have evolved, developed or existed.

So, if you were to ask me if I were to change anything, I know what my answer would be. It's the same answer my mum gives when I ask her if I *really* did *ruin* her life. The answer is yes, *but* I wouldn't have it any other way. And so, I finally get what Mum's meant all these years. The paradox makes sense.

I understand that the very thing that can ruin a life can also make life meaningful and purposeful and make you into a version that you believe to be better.

Of course, I don't know what's next in my life, but what I do know is that I am going to keep living with the death in my body, knowing that it gives me my reason to live.

Paralysis is the death in *her* body that gives *me* life.

I am her, and she *is* me.

I am thirty-six years old and I am eighteen years old.

And now it's time for me to carpe that fucking diem, just as I am.

Acknowledgements

Before I move on to the next chapter of my life and risk forgetting, I will say here and now that writing this book was the most challenging yet most important thing I have ever done.

When my literary agent, Nelle, secured me this opportunity, I was, yet again, at an unexpected crossroads in my life. A dream that I had been chasing for years had just been snatched from me, I was also reeling from the break-up of an abusive relationship, the pandemic was upon us, and my ability to survive was unknown. Then my sore broke down, and I faced months of bed-rest. This book presented me with a lifeline, yet without a clear plan for what I wanted to write, I began to drown in the face of so much adversity.

These are the people who saved me and, therefore, this book.

Mum and Dad, thank you for keeping me safe whilst I struggled my way through this and for encouraging me and empowering me throughout. All children have their parents to thank for giving them life, but very few get that gift twice. Thank you. I dedicate this book to you as I dedicate my life to you.

Bowl, the word 'friend' doesn't encompass what you are to me, nor does friendship come close to defining what we have. You always have been by my side, and I don't believe any single achievement I have detailed in this book – nor the book itself – would have happened had you not given me your strength throughout.

Tom, you may not know this, but you stepped up to help me at the *exact* time I needed you to. Thank you. And as I write this, you are starting your next chapter with Sarah, and I could not be happier for you both. After my crash, you needed an extended family around you, and in her (and all your beautiful friends), you have created the best possible. I love you so much.

Gillian, you were my lifeboat. Just as I began to lose motivation, as the book and bed-rest became too hard to manage, you came to the rescue with the perfect amount of care, compassion and skill.

Caro, pal, we have a way of finding one another when we are most in need, and it happened again. You listened – as only *you* listen – to so much more than the words, and had you not, they would have struggled to make it out of me.

Phoebe, who has been beside me from the earliest moment I can remember, thank you. Your wisdom and your friendship mean everything.

I also want to take this opportunity to write a few more words of thanks and love to those who are in the book but no longer in my life, as well as to those who do not feature in the book but are very much in my life today.

Bone & Soph, let me tell you that I would go through it all again – the crash, the loss, everything – if it meant I got to experience again the level of friendship we once had. I hope this book keeps what we had alive in ways it can no longer be. There could not have been two more extraordinary girls on this earth to have beside me at that time. Thank you.

Jack, I was so fortunate to have shared my body and my life with you. I hope you treasure *her* in your memory, as I do you in mine.

Rory, I'm sorry I happened to you. I am, however, thankful that you happened to me.

Gary, I have tried to find you, but I can't, so if this book does, *thank you.*

Westy, you loved me and treated me better than any man ever has, and although I would never tell you this, you are one of the *most* extraordinary people I have had the privilege of knowing in this life.

Spam, you are *my* fucking Queen, and I too have 'endless words of love and admiration for you'. You are infinitely more than a chapter in my life. You, Bam, are in between the lines of my entire life story.

El, just as your children are my children, your life is my life, and believe me when I say this: our best chapter is yet to come!

Jo, now this chapter is closed, together, we begin the next, and no matter what happens, knowing you will be in all my chapters to come, till the very last, means our life stories will always be the best.

And Dan, thank you for being the friend we all need.

Mag, while you may not be in these pages or still in my life, our chapter together – in Australia and London – will always be one of my absolute favourites.

Dawn, I feel your love and support wherever I go, especially in the way you mother your sister, my mother. She and, therefore, I would be lost without you.

Luca, Harris, Frida and Stella, I hope you all read this one day and understand how much my role as the 'Sara' in your lives means to me.

Sara, each day is fucking 'carpe'd' in your memory. I hope, through this book, that those who never got to know you can, and that you inspire them as much as you inspire everyone who ever had the privilege of knowing you.

Because this book is about my life so far, I feel as though I want to mention and thank everyone who has helped me along the way, but I can't, and besides, once again, it's time; I have *more* extraordinary things to do, places to go and people to meet. Watch out, world, here I come.